A Tapestry
of
Courage

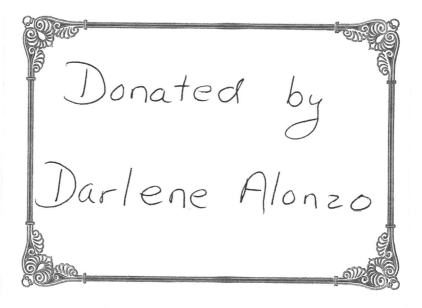

Donated by
Darlene Alonzo

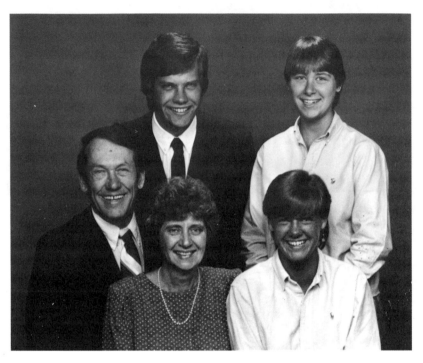

Jimmy, Mary Alice, Katherine, Jim Jr., Mary Ellen

A Tapestry
of
Courage

A Loving Tribute
to Her Daughter

Written by

Mary Alice Welch

ISBN 0-9632509-0-6 (hard cover)
ISBN 0-9632509-1-4 (soft cover)
Library of Congress Catalog Card Number 92-81192

Published by Blue and Gold Publications
Sheffield, MA 01257

Printed by The Studley Press
Dalton, Massachusetts

To Mary Ellen

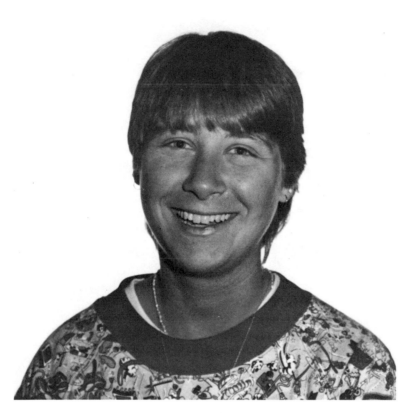

Mary Ellen
1966-1988

"Forever your heart shall beat."

WENDY COOPER PLAISTED
CLASS OF 1989
SPRINGFIELD COLLEGE

v

Acknowledgments

In addition to those who appear in Mary Ellen's story, the following acknowledgments are made with my undying gratitude and affection.

To the teachers, administrators, and staff at Mount Everett Regional School, and Berkshire School, Sheffield, Massachusetts; Springfield College, Springfield, Massachusetts, for their encouragement, support, love and understanding;

To all those employees of Massachusetts Electric Company for their concern and support;

To the doctors, nurses, and staff at Children's Hospital; Brigham and Women's Hospital; The Jimmy Fund Pediatric Clinic of the Dana-Farber Cancer Institute in Boston; the Baystate Medical Center, Springfield, Massachusetts; Sharon Hospital, Sharon, Connecticut; and Hartford Hospital, Hartford, Connecticut for the unfailing care and concern shown Mary Ellen and us;

The Mount Everett Regional School students, in particular my French and Spanish classes, Berkshire School students, and Springfield College students for their unwavering support and love;

Our neighbors, friends, and relatives for always being there for us;

Madeleine L'Engle for her words of encouragement;

Janice Thomas for listening to the tapes and typing the interviews so vital to the completion of this book;

Chris Callahan for his computer expertise and assistance with the intricacies of the computer so generously loaned to me by Jennifer Kinsley;

Dorothy Adams, Leo Alvares, and Marcia Friedman for reading the manuscript and assisting with editing.

Kathie Ness for her very expert, professional assistance.

Most important of all, my gratitude and love to my family— Jimmy, Katherine, and Jim Jr.—without whose understanding, love, and encouragement, I could not have written this book.

Mary Alice Welch

Prologue

In Celebration of the Life of Mary Ellen Welch

I have been asked to give a brief eulogy today, but there are two reasons why I do not intend to do that.

The first reason is that it is impossible. A eulogy is, by tradition, a kind of summary of a person's life, lifting up virtues and highlighting accomplishments. But how can I—or anyone else—even begin to find words to express all that Mary Ellen was and is for us? Think of the range of relationships she had with all of us gathered here today—each relationship different from all the others, each of us sharing a unique level and utterly personal kind of intimacy with her. Some of us saw her as a young woman of incredible strength and courage. Some of us knew her as a human being struggling against fear and doubt. Some of us knew her as an ordinary twenty-two-year-old, full of the delights and frustrations of every young adult. For some of us she was a childhood playmate. For others she was a high school teammate or college classmate or daughter, sister, neighbor, or friend.

In her short life on this small planet, she touched so many of our lives with the gift of her friendship; she wove such a wonderfully intricate tapestry of relationships. And we can only begin to comprehend how vast and far-reaching the fabric of relationships was for Mary Ellen—certainly no words can encompass it. But one thing we can see plainly here today is that as she wove that tapestry of relationships, she not only connected each of us inseparably with herself, but she connected us with one another as well. And because of that, we are all more keenly aware of being part of a larger human family—more sensitive to life, more aware of one another, more able to reach down and draw out the best within our deepest selves. Because of Mary Ellen, we are all more fully human.

The other reason I will not eulogize Mary Ellen is that she would be embarrassed by it. She told some of us last week that she was tired of being—to use her words—"put on a pedestal." She was tired of being hailed as a model of courage and strength of character. She wasn't a hero: she was just an ordinary person who was tired of this awful ordeal, who felt that dying at twenty-two was just plain unfair. I think she was asking if it was okay not to be brave for a while.

Of course, ironically, that was exactly what was so truly heroic about Mary Ellen. She was, in truth, just an ordinary human being like the rest of us. She had strengths and weaknesses, successes and failures, faith and doubt. But this ordinary human being bore her unfair burden with incredible courage and strength of character. And most amazingly, she bore it matter-of-factly, asking no concessions, looking for no special treatment, refusing to fall into the role of playing the martyr. That's why being put up on a pedestal bothered her. She refused to be Mary Ellen the Saint. She just wanted to be Mary Ellen.

I think that was her best gift to us. She lived her life as a simple, ordinary human being who just happened to have a lot to cope with. And in so doing, she showed all the rest of us simple, ordinary human beings that we, too, can cope with whatever burdens we may have to bear in this life. Like Mary Ellen, we, too, can laugh and learn and love in the midst of pain and disappointment. And when our moment to leave this life comes, perhaps we will remember the sense of peace and completion that enveloped her in the end. And we will know that we need not be afraid. What a legacy she has left for us: live life fully, bear our burdens without complaint, greet death peacefully. According to Mary Ellen, that's just living an ordinary life.

One last thought. What happens to us beyond this life is a mystery. Probably all of us envision it a little differently. But that life in some form continues, I am absolutely convinced. It is a basic law of physics that material form can be destroyed, but energy cannot. Energy can only be transformed from one expression to another; it cannot be lost. So, too, with Mary Ellen. Her form may have worn out, but her energy—what is truly Mary Ellen—persists in a new way and in a new realm utterly incomprehensible to us. And although we feel a profound sense of loss, there is also a sense of completion and wondrous new beginning for her. I hope we can all celebrate that.

So, Mary Ellen, thank you for connecting us to you and to one another, and in doing so, helping us to discover a deeper level in ourselves. And thank you for showing us how we ordinary people can face both life and death with courage and humor. You have touched us all; you have helped us on our journeys. Now, Godspeed on yours!

The Rev. Kenneth A. Childs
DIRECTOR OF CAMPUS MINISTRY
SPRINGFIELD COLLEGE
JUNE 14, 1988

Delivered on June 14, 1988, at Our Lady of the Valley Church, Sheffield, Massachusetts at Mary Ellen's funeral.

Part 1

1

🍂

MARY ELLEN'S STORY IS ONE OF COURAGE, DETERMINATION, perseverance, and love. In November of 1982, at age sixteen, Mary Ellen was stricken with osteogenic sarcoma, resulting in the amputation of her right leg. The five and a half years following Mary Ellen's diagnosis were filled with remarkable experiences, reflecting the support of her family, friends, classmates, teachers, and acquaintances. During this time she experienced several thoracotomies, months of chemotherapy treatment, and many radiation treatments. Her story should prove to be an inspiration to those who struggle against seeming insurmountable odds. She may not have won the war, but her battles were hard fought and her courage inspirational. She lived her brief time on this earth to the fullest, leaving behind a legacy of courage and strength.

In 1982, our family—Jimmy and I with our three children, Jim Jr., nineteen, Mary Ellen, sixteen, and Katherine, fifteen—lived in Sheffield, Massachusetts, a small town (population 2,500) located in the very western corner of the state. Jimmy and I had been married for twenty-two years. He worked as a clerk foreman for the Massachusetts Electric Company in Great Barrington and I, since 1971, had taught in the Southern Berkshire Regional School District, based in Sheffield and comprising the towns of New Marlborough, Alford, Sheffield, Monterey, and the Egremonts. Ours was a close-knit family which enjoyed doing things together. Jimmy and I, through our strong Catholic religion, had strived to instill moral and ethical values in our children. We, as a family, were members of Our Lady of the Valley Church in Sheffield, taking an active part in the church community. Jim Jr. had spent a semester at the State University of New York at Cobleskill, leaving there in January 1982, to take a semester to work on a few courses at Berkshire Community College in Pittsfield, Massachusetts, while he was employed in the Outdoor Maintenance Department at the prestigious Red Lion Inn in Stockbridge,

Massachusetts. His major at Cobleskill was in nursery work and landscaping. At this point in his life, we hoped he had stopped growing as he approached a height of 6'3". Mary Ellen, a junior at Mount Everett Regional School, played field hockey, soccer, and softball, and skied during the winter. Mary Ellen tended to be just a bit overweight, or so she thought, and she at times admitted jealousy towards her sister, Katherine, who was quite slim. Mary Ellen was a great supporter of all of the Mount Everett teams, a true Eagle fan. She had quite a sense of humor and loved a crowd. Jesse O'Hara, one of her elementary school teachers, remembers her as a happy, "full of it" fourth grader. Jesse commented, "When the children came in with stories in the morning, she could usually top them."

Katherine, a sophomore at Mount Everett, also participated in softball as well as skiing. Katherine and Mary Ellen each had their own circle of friends at school but usually skied together with their skiing buddies.

The summer of 1982, Veronique Dubes, an exchange student from Bayonne, France, visited us for the month of July. Mary Ellen returned to Bayonne with Veronique and spent three fantastic weeks visiting the Dubes family. When Mary Ellen returned home in August, it was obvious to all of us that she had not taken our advice to watch the calories. She just laughed and said, "The French bread and pâté were delicious." She had probably gained 10 pounds during her three-week stay with the Dubes family. In order to shed this weight, Mary Ellen started running during the last week in August in preparation for the soccer season at Mount Everett.

About the third week in November, Mary Ellen complained of a pain in her right knee. When she was a seventh grader, she had had minor surgery on her left knee for an osteogenic chondroma or osteochondroma, which is a benign type of tumor. This was removed and her leg was fine. She was able to resume her normal routine, particularly skiing, her first love. When she complained now of the pain in her right knee, Jimmy and I thought perhaps it was the same as had occurred previously.

We went to Dr. Joseph Hajek, the orthopedic surgeon at Sharon

Clinic in Sharon, Connecticut, who, after X-raying her knee, told us that he would like a bone scan done immediately. Since we had planned to go to Westchester County, New York, the following day to spend Thanksgiving with our family, Dr. Hajek indicated that the bone scan should be done the first thing the following Monday morning.

The urgency of the bone scan did not penetrate our thoughts as we prepared to spend the holiday visiting my sister, Dolores Viebrock, her family and my parents, Helen and Donald Ward, who lived in Scarsdale, New York. As I prepared my contribution to the Thanksgiving feast, a French apple pie, my thoughts were with our holiday and not with the bone scan.

We loved going to the Viebrock house for the holiday since Dolores is a fantastic cook, always preparing a scrumptious meal. During the day, the cousins watched football and played some touch football and the following day Jimmy and I shopped for Christmas in White Plains.

After the weekend, Mary Ellen and I returned to Sharon Hospital for the bone scan. Dr. Hajek said that we should remain at the hospital until he read the scan. The technician didn't realize this and told us to go home. "Dr. Hajek will call you later today with the results," she said. That evening Dr. Hajek called and said the suspicions he had had when he read the X-ray were confirmed. There was either a tumor or an infection in the base of the femur in Mary Ellen's right leg. He wanted us to come to his office on Wednesday to meet with him and Mary Ellen's pediatrician, Dr. Bill Gallup. He also said that he would make an appointment for Thursday of that week at Children's Hospital in Boston to meet with the head of orthopedics, Dr. Paul Griffin, whom he wanted to verify his findings. When Dr. Hajek told me of the possibility of an amputation, I just couldn't believe it. Jimmy and I talked this over and we decided to wait and see what Wednesday and the meeting with the two doctors would bring before we told Mary Ellen about Dr. Hajek's suspicions.

On Wednesday, when we met with Dr. Gallup and Dr. Hajek, they showed Jimmy and me the pictures of the bone scan and pointed out the area of concern, which could be either an infection or a tumor. I felt they truly thought it was a tumor. The doctors insisted on telling Mary Ellen. However, Jimmy felt she shouldn't know just yet because there was the faint possibility that the amputation would not be necessary. The doctors, on the other hand, said, "We feel we must be honest with you as well as with Mary Ellen. We'll go over the scan with her and tell her our findings." Jimmy, visibly upset because of their decision, could not remain in the office.

The doctors insisted. "We'll speak to Mary Ellen alone if this is all right with you. It might be easier this way." They reviewed the scan and X-rays with her, spoke about Ted Kennedy's amputation, and stressed the need to rid her knee of the tumor or infection, whatever the further tests in Boston showed. After they finished speaking with Mary Ellen, they reminded Jimmy and me of the appointment the following day with Dr. Griffin. We gathered together the X-rays and other papers to present to Dr. Griffin and soberly left the clinic offices.

The ride home was a quiet one. No one seemed to have anything to say, as we were wrapped up in our own thoughts about this meeting. At home I was starting to prepare dinner when Mary Ellen came into the kitchen and asked me, "What exactly did Dr. Gallup and Dr. Hajek mean?" She really had not understood the full impact of their discussion. Who could blame her? The farthest thing from anyone's mind would be the loss of a limb. I had to tell her then that there was the possibility of an infection or of a tumor, which would perhaps result in the amputation of her right leg. Horrified as my words suddenly took on meaning, Mary Ellen began to sob.

As I comforted her, I said, "We're not sure that the worst is going to happen. Let's wait until we meet with the doctor at Children's before we start to think the worst." This we did.

2
❦

THE NEXT DAY WE FOUND OUR WAY TO CHILDREN'S HOSPITAL, after getting lost in downtown Boston. We met with an assistant of Dr. Griffin's and Mary Ellen was admitted. As we went up the elevator to the sixth floor, little did we know that this would be our home away from home for the next five and a half years. In a few short days our relatively uncomplicated lives had become filled with apprehension and fear. We were familiar with Ted Kennedy's story, and Mary Ellen and Katherine had seen him skiing at Butternut Basin, the ski area in Great Barrington where they skied every winter weekend. Ted and his family were friends of the Murdocks, who owned Butternut, and often skied there during vacations. But we never dreamed that this disease could happen to one of our children.

Jimmy and I were both of the same mind when it came to our children. They came first—not that they were spoiled or catered to, but they were our reasons for being. Vacations—whether they were fall weekends at a ranch in Lake George, weeks at Cape Cod in the summer, or weekend skiing trips to Vermont—were family affairs. We grew together, planning most of our activities around our family. The kids were very rarely sick—a sore throat or cold periodically was the extent of their illnesses. Visits to the pediatrician were infrequent. We watched them grow from babies to teenagers, experiencing the usual sibling rivalry and arguments. Far from being perfect, they were, however, good kids who, we hoped and prayed, would develop strong moral characters as they continued into their teenage years. Because of our strong faith in God, I believe that we received strength from Him to cope with what the future had in store for us as a family. As we began what would prove to be a five-and-a-half-year battle, we had the support of one another and our children; three of the best kids in the world fighting together with us to maintain a normal lifestyle whenever possible. For this would be the route we would take—

following our already established pattern of a close-knit family helping one another to deal with any and all trials that would arise.

3
❦

UPON OUR ARRIVAL ON DIVISION 26, THE SIXTH-FLOOR PEDI-atric orthopedic center at Children's Hospital, Mary Ellen was given her bed and settled in by her nurses, Jen and Debbie. Jimmy and I went to the cafeteria for a quick supper, hoping to be back when the doctors made their rounds. When Jen came to the cafeteria to tell us of their arrival, we hurriedly returned to Division 26 to find an entourage of medical people—Dr. John Emans, orthopedic surgeon of the osteogenic team; his resident, Dr. Mark Gebhart; Dr. Alan Goorin of the Jimmy Fund Pediatric Clinic of the Dana-Farber Cancer Institute,* head of the osteogenic sarcoma protocol (the plan for chemotherapy treatments); and Dr. Eva Guinan, an oncology fellow (a doctor who treats cancer patients) associated with the Pediatric Clinic. Dr. Emans outlined the situation with Mary Ellen and us. The problem was a tumor at the base of the femur in the right leg. Osteogenic sarcoma was the diagnosis. This disease can strike ages ten to twenty-five and there are approximately 900 cases a year in the United States. At the time that Mary Ellen was stricken, statistics indicated that 60 percent of

---

* The Dana-Farber, founded in 1975 as the Children's Cancer Research Foundation, is the world's first organization devoted exclusively to childhood cancer research and treatment. In 1948 the Boston Braves baseball team "adopted" a little boy named Jimmy, who was a cancer patient at the Dana-Farber. His struggle became a team effort, as from all across America donations were sent to Boston. The Jimmy Fund came into being and has, at present, raised millions of dollars to support cancer research and the care of children with cancer. Children under the age of eighteen may be cared for in the Jimmy Fund Clinic.

cases went into remission (disease-free survival with no relapse for five years) with an overall survival rate of 75 percent.

Dr. Emans directed his comments primarily toward Mary Ellen because, as he said, "She's sixteen—and she will have to make the decision regarding the options given. It's her leg."

What a decision to have to make at age sixteen! Decisions at this age were supposed to be "Should I or shouldn't I cut my hair? Wear a skirt or jeans? Go to the dance or to the movies? Go skiing or snowmobiling?" Why should a sixteen-year-old girl have to make such a dreadful decision? Why indeed? This was to be only the first of many major decisions Mary Ellen would make with us during the next five years.

The medical staff outlined the plan. The following Tuesday, December 7, Dr. Emans would perform a biopsy. If the biopsy verified his suspicions, he would continue with the option that Mary Ellen chose from the four options he gave her. The first option was to do nothing. This, of course, was out of the question as far as we all were concerned. We wanted to rid her leg of this cancerous tumor as soon as possible so she could get on with her life. The next was the amputation. Her right leg would be amputated above the knee, thus getting rid of the tumor and leaving as much of a residual limb as possible so a prosthesis would fit really well. The third option was a rather weird arrangement called a turn-about. The knee joint, as well as portions of the leg above and below the knee, are resected (cut away). Then the ankle section is turned backwards and reattached to the thigh area so that the ankle can function as a knee joint. Mary Ellen wasn't happy about a solution such as this. She did talk with a young man, Joey Race, who had elected to have a turn-about. He chose it because he felt he would have the mobility to roller skate. The fourth option would be a resection to remove the tumor, keeping the leg. A rod would be inserted in the leg and there would perhaps be periodic visits to surgery with this solution, as well as very little mobility. She would not be able to run, to ski, to play softball—to do all those activities that she had been used to doing.

Dr. Emans therefore asked, "Just what exactly do you want to be able to do after the tumor is removed?"

9

Mary Ellen answered, "I want to be able to do just about what I've been doing. I don't want to sit on my fanny and not take part in some athletics."

Dr. Emans responded, "The amputation and then a good-fitting prosthesis will give you the most mobility. You'll be able to ski with outriggers and you'll probably be able to play some sports."

That evening, after the discussion, Mary Ellen decided upon the amputation.

After the decision, the oncologists on the team, Dr. Goorin and Dr. Guinan, told us of the part they would be playing. They would monitor Mary Ellen's progress through Dr. Emans. After the operation, we would meet with them to discuss fully the protocol to be followed. At this point, Dr. Goorin and Dr. Guinan spoke about a randomization that was in effect for osteogenic sarcoma. This plan, as the term indicates, meant that some patients might elect the chemotherapy protocol of thirteen months or they might elect no treatment at the time of amputation. The randomization was a study begun at St. Jude's Medical Center in Tennessee with the National Cancer Institute. The study compared the two groups—one the chemo group and the other the non-chemo group. If, however, any of the patients relapsed while in the non-chemo group, treatments would begin immediately. The study thus far had shown that 40 percent of the patients in the non-chemo group were disease-free.

Again, Mary Ellen had a major decision to make, not immediately, but within the next two weeks. We discussed the randomization at length, but we wanted any decision to be hers. However, I did call Dr. Gallup, explaining the dilemma to him. If Mary Ellen chose the chemo, the side effects could prove life-threatening. But were she to choose the non-chemo group, the cells might metastasize very quickly, causing some very serious problems with her lungs. After speaking with Dr. Gallup, we decided to do as he suggested: "I'd go for all the protection they could afford." So Mary Ellen made another decision—to go with the chemotherapy protocol.

4

❦

JIMMY AND I STAYED AT NEARBY MOTELS WHILE MARY ELLEN spent those first few days in the hospital. We had searched out inexpensive places, realizing that this might be a long confinement. Our meals could be taken at the hospital, but paying for motels would take a big chunk of our savings. While Mary Ellen was a patient on Division 26 for those first few days, we met Johanna and Roy Rinkle, whose daughter, Pia, was being treated for a serious leg infection. Johanna and I, both feeling the need to communicate as we sat with our children, became friends. She knew we were having difficulties finding reasonable places to stay. We had investigated the Ronald McDonald House, but there was no room those first few days. Perhaps had we really kept after the social services department at the hospital, we would have found a place. My sister, who has three children who worked for McDonald's in Hawthorne, New York, called the manager of the Hawthorne Restaurant, who in turn contacted someone else. Dolores called us one day to say, "There's a room available for you today if you need one."

In the meantime, however, Johanna and Roy offered us the use of an apartment in their rather large home in Newton, about twenty minutes from the hospital. We were completely overwhelmed by their generosity.

This was the beginning of a long battle—five and a half years—but it was also the beginning of an outpouring of help and kindness that we experienced throughout this entire struggle. Our neighbors in Sheffield and the surrounding towns, our relatives, the schools and colleges Mary Ellen attended, friends and classmates—just about everyone with whom she came in contact—came to our assistance. We learned a very valuable lesson: one does not have to struggle alone. We learned the true meaning of friendship, beginning with our meeting Johanna and Roy Rinkle. We know now that we could not have coped by ourselves. We accepted the offers of our friends and of new acquaintances, who over these years have become friends. To realize that we did not have to face the ups and downs alone was very comforting. The outpouring of love and concern in a true Christian spirit helped us to go from day to day, knowing that a helping hand was only a phone call away.

The threads to weave Mary Ellen's tapestry were prepared on the loom as the impending seriousness of the disease consumed our every thought and word. Through the years until June 1988, the weaving of colors, personalities, and events would result in a tapestry, the threads of which would intertwine, mesh, and blend, depicting Mary Ellen's journey as she, as well as we, her family, experienced a remarkable five and a half years. The threads ultimately wove with texture and dimension this tapestry of courage in which all of her friends and acquaintances shared in her short life, and enriched ours. Today, many of these individuals experience a more positive outlook and a profound love of life because of their relationship with Mary Ellen.

5
❧

AFTER THE TESTS AND OTHER MEDICAL DECISIONS WERE MADE, and after Jimmy and I had settled into the Rinkle's apartment, the doctors indicated that Mary Ellen could go home on Saturday, only to return the next day in order to get ready for the operation on Tuesday, December 7. We were delighted to be able to go home, even if only overnight; but with the homecoming was the task of telling our family and friends the devastating news.

A very difficult phone call to make was the one to my parents, telling them of the outcome of the tests. My mother suffered from arthritis, which had debilitated her almost to the point of rendering her an invalid. My father had retired from his position as a senior officer of Kidder, Peabody, Inc., and took care of her. They were crushed by our news, and their reaction, along with that of our aunts and uncles, was, "Why did this have to happen to such a young girl? Why not to one of us? We've lived our lives and she's only beginning hers." The prayers offered by these concerned relatives, I'm sure, helped to give us the strength to carry on.

When we arrived home, Katherine met us at the door. She had done all of the washing and had just finished the ironing. These chores were not usually part of Katherine's routine, but this was her way of making things easier for all of us. What could we say? The die was cast, so to speak, and Katherine and Jim Jr. would cope along with Mary Ellen, Jimmy, and me. We told them of the plans for the operation and that we would be returning to Children's Hospital Sunday afternoon, with the operation to take place on December 7. We all decided that they should remain home, going to school and work, while Jimmy and I returned with Mary Ellen. There were many offers for dinners, especially from Katherine's friend Jennifer's family, the Kinsleys. Sue Kinsley made a delicious spaghetti dinner for us upon our arrival home and could be counted upon to see that Jim Jr. and his sister would be well taken care of while we were in Boston.

Saturday evening Mary Ellen telephoned many friends, inviting them for lunch on Sunday before we had to return to Boston. We had a picnic with hamburgers and all the trimmings as she told her friends what would be in store for her these next few days. As I reflect upon those days, I marvel at Mary Ellen's composure as she told her dear friends and others about the amputation. I know God in His infinite wisdom and caring was setting the stage for the battle by giving each of us the grace to deal with this affliction. Mary Ellen particulary was in command as she told her friends exactly what was going to transpire. "But don't worry," she said, as she wore her infectious smile, "I'll have a prosthesis and I'll be able to do just about everything I'm doing now." In spite of the terrible ordeal that she was going to face, she managed to make her friends and us feel better because of her incredibly optimistic outlook.

6

SUNDAY AFTERNOON JIMMY, MARY ELLEN, AND I RETURNED to Boston and the hospital. The following day there were more tests, more discussions, and more nurses and others to meet. One of these was Shelley Goverman, who became Mary Ellen's primary care physical therapist. Shelley has since indicated to me that her first meeting with Mary Ellen was a bit different from her other cases, since she had to deal with a patient who had not lost her leg and had no physical problem as yet. But as Shelley said, "There I was. I had to evaluate her, to educate her. I wasn't sure if I should ignore the leg entirely or what the story was."

And then Mary Ellen was very casual as she said, "This is the one that's coming off."

"She was pretty cheerful and straightforward right from the start. We chatted and found out that I knew someone who had married a young man whom you all knew from the neighboring town of Alford. So right from the start we really hit it off."

Ellen Z (we used her last initial since there was another Ellen on the floor) and Beth, two nurses from Division 36, the adolescent orthopedic area, came to visit and to introduce themselves to us and to Mary Ellen. After the amputation, Mary Ellen would be a patient on Division 36, where Ellen Z would be her primary care nurse.

It was during this day that an X-ray indicated that there might be tumors in Mary Ellen's lungs. Since this cancer is characterized by metastases to the lungs, and since all precautions were to be taken, the doctors decided that a thoracotomy* would be performed on December 9, two days after the amputation. Now we were faced with the thought of two major surgeries in two days.

---

* A thoracotomy is the removal of tumors or metastases from the lung by taking a section or piece of the lung surrounding the tumor(s) to ensure, if posible, the removal of possible cancer cells along with tumor(s).

Everything was happening so quickly that we didn't have time to dwell on all that we had been told. This in itself was, I feel, a blessing because with little time to think about our situation, we were better able to cope with each day.

As the day ended and we were getting ready to return to the apartment, we told Mary Ellen that we would be glad to stay with her during the night. But she characteristically said, "No. You guys go home and get some sleep. I'll be fine. I'll see you in the morning, early." We assured her we would be there before she went down to the operating room and then, giving her some kisses and hugs, we went off to try to relax in preparation for the next day.

About nine o'clock her nurse, Jen, called. "Could you come back to the hospital? Mary Ellen really wants to see you."

We quickly drove to the hospital to find Mary Ellen scared and nervous. She hated to bother us to return to the hospital, but she was considerably upset and just wanted to be with us. We assured her again that we'd stay the night if she wanted us to.

"No," she said. "I just wanted to talk with you." We sat with her and talked to her and prayed with her.

I reminded Mary Ellen of a dear friend, Wendy Smith, who had died two years before and who had shared many activities with Mary Ellen at Mount Everett. I said, "I know Wendy is with you during this difficult time and I'm certain she will ask Our Blessed Lady to watch over you and to take care of you during the operation and afterward. And when the operation is over, Our Lady will continue to be there for you."

After a little while, she said she felt better and could now go to sleep. She again told us, "Go home."

"Remember," we said, "we're only a phone call away."

Jen reassured us, "I'll call you no matter the time if she wants you."

I believe sincerely that Our Blessed Lady did hear our prayers and from that point on in our struggle, Mary Ellen became very special to her and to her Son. I recall a priest stating once, "Those who suffer are closest to God." I knew that the strength we all needed to pull together to get through this ordeal would come from His grace. He would not let us down. I know, therefore, in my heart and soul that from that day on, Mary Ellen was under the protection of Our Lady's mantle. I recall the day of Mary Ellen's baptism. The reason we named her Mary Ellen was that she was born on the feast of the Annunciation of our Blessed Lady, March 25th.

After the Baptism, we carried her to the side altar, to the statue of Our Lady where Father Edmund Healey, our pastor, dedicated Mary Ellen to our Blessed Lady, invoking her protection. I know that no one could experience what we did as a family without receiving the grace to endure from Our Lord, Jesus Christ, through the intercession of His Mother.

An insight in regard to the meaning of her name was revealed on a beautifully printed card she received from Benjamin Dubes, Veronique's brother, after the trip to France.

Marie signifie "illuminatrice" et Hélène "éclat de soleil." Gracieuses et élégantes, les Marie. Hélène brillent et dominent dès qu'elles sont en société, tout en restant très sympathiques.

The French have such a beautiful way of expressing thoughts. The English translation isn't quite so poetic, but the meaning in whatever language certainly is appropriate.

Mary means "one who lights" and Ellen a "burst of sunshine." Marys are gracious and elegant. Ellens shine and dominate while they are with people, all the time remaining very nice.

As we left the hospital again and drove back to the apartment, I thought, "It's no wonder she can't sleep. The apprehension overwhelmed us and her." During these past five days, we talked about the tests, consultations, doctors' visits, and the final outcome—the amputation. We wanted to be rid of this awful tumor. Mary Ellen had accepted the idea of the prosthesis, especially since the medical people indicated she would have very little difficulty becoming accustomed to it. Dr. Emans said he would be able to leave a good residual limb to insure a proper fit for the prosthesis. As the night moved closer to daylight, Jimmy and I accepted the inevitable as we awaited the morning and surgery.

7

IN THE EARLY MORNING WE AGAIN DROVE IN FROM THE RINKLES', arriving at the hospital about 7 p.m. We hurried through the lobby, at this hour silent and almost eerie without the usual hustle or bustle. On the sixth floor, as we walked down the darkened hallway to Mary Ellen's room, we noted the only activity to be a group of residents and interns making rounds and one or two nurses walking quickly in and out of the patients' rooms, their voices hushed as the children slept. Breakfast trays were not due for another hour.

Mary Ellen was dozing, having been given medication. Our niece, Maureen Ward, joined us as we awaited the operating room escort to transport Mary Ellen to the operating room on the third floor. Maureen, a student at Fisher Junior College in Boston, just happened to be doing an internship in the activity room at Children's on Division 26. She had visited Mary Ellen several times during the few days she was hospitalized and was great company. Maureen had planned to pursue a career similar to her internship at the hospital. A few months after Mary Ellen's operation, Maureen admitted to Jimmy, "I became too involved with Mary Ellen's illness and realized that if I pursued my present goals, I would be coming in contact with many very ill young people. Right there and then I decided that I would have to change my goals and look for a position working with young people outside the hospital scene." During the next five and a half years, Mary Ellen would come in contact with several people who would feel her presence and who would look to her for guidance and assistance.

Soon the operating room escort, Danny Tucker, arrived and Mary Ellen, with Jimmy, Maureen, and me, began her journey down the elevator to the third floor and the pre-op holding room, where we awaited the signal from the team that all was ready. Mary Ellen, having been sedated, was sleepy and did not see our tears of anguish. We still hoped for that tiny ray of light; maybe the

17

biopsy that Dr. Emans planned to do first would indicate a non-malignant tumor with no need for the drastic amputation. Deep down we had resigned ourselves to the bitter fact, but even so, we still could hope until the biopsy was final. The nurses told us that all was ready as they wheeled Mary Ellen toward the dreaded double doors of the OR.

We were not forgotten as the nurses said, "Go downstairs to the cafeteria and have some breakfast. By then the liaison nurse in the parents' waiting area in the lobby will have word about the nature of the biopsy." We kissed Mary Ellen goodbye and the three of us tearfully made our way to the cafeteria.

After we had had a bite to eat and some coffee, we reported to the liaison nurse, whose job was to keep parents informed about the activity in the operating room. In a short while she reported to us that the biopsy had been done and the results were as suspected. Dr. Emans would amputate Mary Ellen's right leg. We would be kept informed and updated. All we could do now was to sit, to pray, and to wait.

In what seemed like an eternity but was probably about two or three hours, we received a report from Dr. Emans that all had gone as hoped and that Mary Ellen would soon be in her room on Division 36. We could go upstairs and wait for her. The Division 36 nurses were well versed in caring for osteogenic patients and were very skillful in administering the chemotherapy necessary. Again we met Ellen Z who would be Mary Ellen's primary care nurse for as long as she was a patient on Division 36. Kathi Kelly, Mary Beth, Coolie, Putney, and Ruth—to name a few—would be her nurses during the many months ahead.

Mary Ellen returned to the room, still groggy from the anesthesia. As we waited for her to awaken, a young girl in one of the other beds asked, "What's the matter with her?" We explained about the surgery. A young friend who was visiting couldn't believe his ears. He walked over to Mary Ellen's bed, eyes wide, and stared for a brief moment, shaking his head in disbelief.

Now that this surgery was completed, we hoped that all would move along smoothly. We knew the results of the upcoming surgery to remove the two tiny tumors in her lungs might be ominous, but again we hoped they would not be metastases. Mary Ellen, we felt, would progress through recovery and the upcoming chemotherapy protocol with no major problems. The diagnosis, hospitalization, and amputation took place in a week's time, so we had little opportunity to really dwell on these events. Our thoughts now turned to getting Mary Ellen back on the road to recovery so she could resume her everyday routine.

Our reactions, as well as hers, to the events of the last week were difficult to sort out. We were devastated that Mary Ellen had to suffer through this ordeal; however, as we became acquainted with the hospital and the patients, we realized that there were other children and young people who were very much worse off than Mary Ellen. We were a family that would deal with this together, supporting her every inch of the way. I know that Mary Ellen was as devastated as we were, but it was not in her nature to feel sorry for herself. So as she recovered in the hospital, we thought ahead to the good times when all this would be behind us and she would resume all of her activities. Mary Ellen accepted the situation and four years later, as a freshman at Springfield College in 1986, she remarked at a dinner as the guest speaker of the American Cancer Society, "It's a bummer, but it happened and I can't change anything. The only thing I can do is look toward the future with a positive attitude."

Look toward the future she did. When life with only one leg began in 1982, Mary Ellen accepted her fate and from then on set an example of courage, determination, and perseverance that was indeed inspiring. She never wanted to be looked upon as "different" and never wanted to be treated differently from all the other kids. She continued doing the usual teenage activities, only varying her routine when chemo, radiation, or surgery intervened. These she treated as temporary setbacks, squeezing them into her life and, as soon as they were out of the way, continuing to do her thing.

I remember many a time driving home from Boston after a lengthy treatment and Mary Ellen asking, "Is there a game today?" If there were one, she'd demand to be dropped off at school instead of going home. She could have been confined to bed or the wheelchair with the IV for anywhere from four to six days, but once she left the hospital and that particular treatment was over, she'd bounce back to being her old self—despite the fact that she had probably spent most of the hospital stay "puking her guts out." We used to marvel at her, as did others. She would immediately turn off the cancer part of her life after the treatment was finished and resume all of her regular activities until it was time for the next treatment or monthly hospital check. We would say that Mary Ellen put on her "Boston face" as each treatment day approached.

It was miraculous, this strength and courage she had. I truly feel her strength was also transferred to us because we, too, became strong. We coped. We knew we had to because we could not let her see how devastated we were. Therefore, I know that God gave us all that special grace to meet this challenge head-on and to carry on our daily routines with a smile.

From the beginning of her struggle until the end of the battle— June 1988—Mary Ellen became the embodiment of strength and courage for many. An acquaintance, Duchee Vining, who is also a physical therapist by profession, writes of the profound effect Mary Ellen's amputation had upon her.

> *I didn't know Mary Ellen except from afar, and I don't think she would have known me even to say 'Hello.' But, like many others, I had to follow her progress and struggles from a distance and was impressed and inspired by her. Without knowing her, I learned a lot from her.*
>
> *I can picture clearly Jeannette Cooper telling me of the need for her amputation, and I remember clearly sitting at my piano at the hour of her surgery, sadly plunking out a few notes and thinking of her and of one of the first patients I had as a student physical therapist at Children's Hospital. Her name was Maureen Cahill, she was about sixteen, and she had recently had a lower limb amputation because of bone cancer. She was only a few years younger than I was. As much as I tried to understand her, relate to her, and befriend her, I sadly realized at the time of Mary Ellen's surgery that I had thought of Maureen as a patient and an amputee and had neglected to think of who she was before she became ill and what the process of her illness and surgery had meant. Knowing of your family and of Mary Ellen before her illness and thinking of your experiences that day was a real growth experience for*

*me, and I hope that both personally and professionally my contacts with
others will be enhanced by that.*

*I don't think I ever saw Mary Ellen when she didn't have a smile on
her face and a crowd of friends and family around her. You didn't have
to know her to be affected by her charisma. It showed during her illness;
and the image of a cane, a bandanna, and a perpetual smile I'm sure
will long give many people the courage to continue on in the face of
adversities. Many people were inspired by her and were rooting for her,
and many lost much the day the battle ended. That she touched so many
lives in a positive sense was surely some measure of the special person
Mary Ellen was.*

After the amputation, when Jim Jr. and Katherine visited Mary
Ellen, I'm certain they were apprehensive. "What do we say?"
"What do we do?" These questions were going around in their
thoughts. When they arrived at Mary Ellen's room, she greeted
them with "Do you want to see?" At this point, it was certainly
understandable that neither wanted to look at the results of the
operation. In fact, Mary Ellen spoke about their apprehension to
Shelley Goverman, saying "They couldn't deal with it." During
their visit, Mary Ellen smiled, talked, and enjoyed their company.
She put them at ease, for she had a knack for doing this. Soon we
were all talking and laughing as she introduced her brother and
sister to the other girls in the room and to everyone else who
entered. Because of her attitude, I know that Jim and Katherine
felt more relaxed upon leaving than they had ever supposed they
would.

Jim Jr. was an extremely sensitive young man who did not
verbalize as much as his two sisters. During the first part of the
protocol, we counted on him to be our chauffeur and companion
for many Boston trips and for the inevitable blood tests. Often
after a disappointing clinic visit he would question, "Mary Ellen's
going to be all right, isn't she?" During one chemo treatment early
on in the protocol, Jim Jr. and I were with Mary Ellen in the
hospital when she expressed the desire for a fish filet from
McDonald's. We would do anything to encourage her to eat, so
Jim left the hospital, ran the three blocks to McDonald's, and
returned with a still-hot fish filet. We were delighted Mary Ellen

21

had shown an interest in food! However, after the first bite, she remarked, "I guess I'm not really that hungry." Jim Jr. proceeded to finish the fish filet.

Katherine had a very close relationship with Mary Ellen. She continued to be attentive to her sister and often included Mary Ellen in her plans. They loved to shop, go to the movies, to Friendly's, and when Mary Ellen was able, to ski.

These first few days we survived primarily because of Mary Ellen's positive outlook and also because of all the prayers, letters, flowers, and gifts. The cards poured in, and as they did, I made a vow to send cards whenever I heard of someone ill because these remembrances certainly picked up her siprits. Jo Langer's first grade class at Sheffield Center School sent Mary Ellen handmade cards with the note "I hope you'll be better soon." All the classes at Mount Everett signed huge cards, many handmade and forwarded in boxes and large, intriguing envelopes. Everyone remembered her, especially those of the Mount Everett family. Marcia Brolli, an English teacher at Mount Everett, seemed to echo the thoughts and feelings of all when she wrote:

Dear Mary Ellen,
Perhaps you know how much you and your family are loved back here in the "sticks." It's unfortunate you have to learn this now, when a swelled head is going to add to your problems. However, the affection is real, and your infliction (swelled head) will get worse when we thank you for being the catalyst which has brought the whole school together. The family that is Mount Everett is alive and well and "cooking with gas."

There was so much mail from the Berkshires that the nurses kept repeating, "Are you sure all of these towns are in Massachusetts? We've never heard of them." They couldn't get over the postmarks—Sheffield, Mill River, Great Barrington, Housatonic, North Egremont, South Egremont, Ashley Falls. We often commented, "Yes, there's life west of Worcester."

22

8
❦

Two days after the amputation, Mary Ellen went to the third floor again as the surgeon Dr. David Tapper performed a thoracotomy to remove what had been observed on the X-ray and what we hoped would prove to be nothing—no metastases. After this operation, Mary Ellen went to the intensive care unit for twenty-four hours. As Jimmy and I arrived at the ICU after she had been settled, I thought, "This is real. This is what operations are all about." She was hooked up to the monitors, with chest tubes leading to a suction-type apparatus by the bed. She looked so vulnerable, so still. The unit was arranged in such a way that each bed had its own area with machines and devices to monitor the patient. One nurse was assigned to two units. Many of the nurses wore clogs, as did the doctors in the operating room. When we asked why, they indicated they were more comfortable than regular shoes, especially since they spent the greater part of their working day on their feet.

We spent much of the day with Mary Ellen as we waited for her to awaken and to recognize us. Shelley came to visit, as did some of the nurses from Division 36, where Mary Ellen would go the next day. As she remained sleepy and groggy, we left in the early evening. When we returned the next morning, she was back on Division 36.

Now we awaited the pathology report regarding the objects removed from her lungs. Finally, much to our relief and joy, the report indicated that they were not malignant tumors resulting from metastases but rather hard little objects that one might find in the lungs of those who breathe unclear air. We stated to all, "There's nothing purer than Berkshire air." However, since osteogenic sarcoma is characterized by metastases to the lungs, Mary Ellen would be subject to an X-ray each month as a precaution.

As Mary Ellen healed from the thoracotomy, Shelley's work

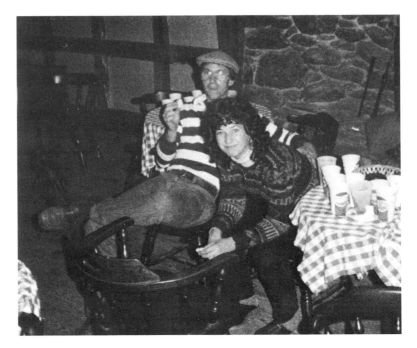

Barnett and Shelley

began in earnest. Not only was Shelley to work with Mary Ellen as a therapist, but she and her husband, Barnett, also became good friends whom we learned to depend upon during our struggle. During lighter times, Shelley and Barnett introduced our taste buds to Chinese cuisine. They thought it incredible that up until our acquaintance with Boston, we had never experienced "Chinese." Despite the very close friendship that developed between Shelley and Mary Ellen, Shelley maintained a strong professional attitude geared to improving Mary Ellen's use of her prosthesis and to keeping her aware of the need for physical exercise. Throughout the years, Shelley was totally committed to helping Mary Ellen develop strength in both limbs—her whole leg and her stump.

After Mary Ellen's death, Shelley discussed her initial visits to Mary Ellen as she recovered from the surgeries. Shelley stated: "Mary Ellen had the chest tubes as I transferred her from the bed to the chair the first or second day after surgery. Since she didn't get a temporary prosthesis, she had such a hard time shrinking. It may have been a philosophical decision not to have a temporary done right then, perhaps because of the thoracotomy." The basic premise for this temporary prosthesis, a cast with a post attached to best simulate a leg, is so the patient starts to walk with a prosthetic gait immediately and the stump starts to shrink rapidly. Since this was not done at the time of amputation, Shelley worked with Mary Ellen, helping her to become accustomed to using crutches before she went home on December 16. Mary Ellen had experienced using crutches previously when she recovered from the surgery on her left knee a few years back so she was an apt pupil. The physical therapy gym on the sixth floor was their classroom. Shelley made arrangements for the fitting of a temporary prosthesis when we returned on December 21.

Besides working with Shelley in the gym, Mary Ellen and I had to learn how to "wrap" her stump, using three 3-inch Ace bandages. The wrapping process would continue forever, since it helped to keep the limb in a controlled position during the night, ensuring a good prosthetic fit. Since Mary Ellen did not receive any type of cast immediately after the surgery, her stump did not shrink and increased post-op swelling resulted. Wrapping was of the utmost importance therefore.

I began wrapping her stump as Mary Ellen requested. I didn't mind doing this for her, and at first it was easier for me to do the wrapping. However, as the weeks went on and I was still wrapping, Shelley became a bit dismayed. She kept urging Mary Ellen to perform this task for herself, but Mary Ellen continued to want me to do it. After Mary Ellen died, Shelley and I talked about the reasons behind her refusal to wrap. We came to the conclusion that this was perhaps her way of showing a need for some dependence. She had been doing well in other areas, but maybe she just felt she didn't want to be completely and totally independent. In every other area she was her own person, able to carry on at school, to go out socially to the movies and school dances. Perhaps this was her way of not wanting to become completely and totally independent, carrying on by herself. She perhaps needed this link with us.

Mary Ellen was discharged December 16, and we happily said our goodbyes as we were reminded to return December 21 for the prosthesis. Ann Carlson, one of Mary Ellen's nurses, affectionately known as Coolie, remembers the departure with the smiles and cheery farewells: "Goodbye, Coolie, I'm going to miss you."

Coolie noted, "As I said goodbye to her, leaving with the flowers, balloons, and stuffed animals, I knew what she had in front of her—the thirteen-month-long chemo protocol. I knew I would be seeing a great deal more of her." Coolie continued, "I remember taking care of her a lot. I remember her being just your regular kid, just like the cheerleader. I think I was taken by just how well she accepted the amputation."

9

❦

THE NEXT DAY, MARY ELLEN PLANNED TO VISIT MOUNT Everett for a Spirits Works Assembly. The word had spread that she had returned home from Boston, a bit earlier than we had thought possible, in a way disappointing her classmates who were planning a "safari" to Boston to spend the weekend cheering up Mary Ellen. During this day, beginning with the arrival of the buses in the morning and continuing through the entire day, Mark Raskind, a math teacher, and two friends, Kurt Callahan and Dave Gauthier, planned to videotape all activities and to send the tape to Mary Ellen. It was a great idea and we arrived in time to appear on the tape as they videoed the assembly.

Mount Everett principal Raymond Chamberland recalls this day, as his thoughts then were filled with mixed emotions.

The Mount Everett family has had its share of sorrow with many student deaths through its short history. The Sunday morning when Mel's aunt, Lorraine Ward, informed me of the impending amputation, I could not cope. Tears, rage, and hate. Why us again? Why me to handle the trauma? Almost forgotten was that nice kid, Mel, with the everyday greeting, 'Hi, Mr. C.'

Then December 17 and the assembly arrived. Mel's mom told me Mel was looking forward to being there, since she would be home from the hospital December 16. My immediate reaction was: Who needs this kind of sorrow at Christmas time? We're trying to turn an attitude around with our "Renew" theme and now we're going to have a "downer."

Assembly day came with spirits high, as was my anxiety. Then Mel arrived; thin, managing crutches, without one of her appendages, but God bless her with that same smile, only brighter, and now her greeting was not just, 'Hi, Mr. C,' but 'Hi world! Come out and look me over!'

To me, Mount Everett changed that day. We greeted Mel not with pity but with family love. She was ours. She became our leader that day. She lifted us to new heights as we began to soar. We all—staff, students, and community—knew nothing could stop us now.

I shall never forget that child who came to lead us and, as the beautiful Catholic hymn says, 'To lift us up on eagles' wings.'

As we entered the gym, Mary Ellen was delighted to see her friends: Danielle Cote, Lisa Gulotta, Ronwyn Ives, Hannah Pedersen, Kurt Callahan, Duane Lanoue, Laurie Briggs, and Denise Sadera. The faculty and the staff were also on hand to give her her first "standing ovation." Being a gregarious young lady, not shy or timid, Mary Ellen knew everyone and acknowledged all with her infectious smile. She grew to love these "Standing O's"—whether the occasion was a softball banquet at Mount Everett, a sports assembly and graduation at Berkshire School, or a meeting of the American Cancer Society.

A huge white sheet, colorfully decorated by Danielle with the message, "Welcome back, Mel," hung on the gym wall. Her friends presented her with an impressively large white teddy bear. Bears were her favorite stuffed animals and during the years she accumulated a small army of them, all sizes and all endearing. One day after her death I spotted a bumper sticker which would have made her day. It said, "Teddy lovers know how to grin and bear it." Maybe Mel knew this all along, thus explaining her affinity for bears.

Prior to the assembly, Danielle, Mary Ellen's longtime friend—

whom she first met at age four when both girls attended the same play group and who became an important part in all our lives— voiced her concern as she said, "I don't think I can handle seeing Mary Ellen and talking to her."

"Danielle," I said, "you above all of the others here at Mount Everett will handle the situation and will continue to be her close friend."

During the next few years, Mary Ellen and Danielle shared many an adventure, sad ones as well as happy ones. The culmination of their friendship was April 27, 1987, when Mary Ellen proudly walked down the aisle as the maid of honor in Danielle's wedding.

During the assembly, Danielle later told me, some of the kids who were more or less "in charge" of the eventual gift-giving indicated that Danielle shouldn't be involved in the ceremony since she and Mary Ellen weren't "hanging out" together as much as the other kids. They attempted to shut Danielle out, trying to monopolize the event and Mary Ellen. These schoolmates meant

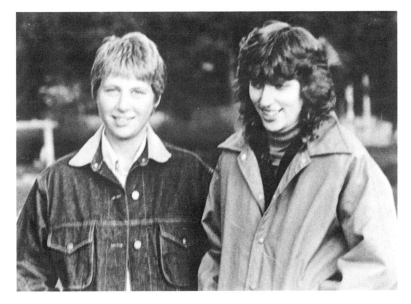

Mary Ellen and Danielle

well, but as time would tell, the novelty, as Danielle so aptly said, "wore off." Danielle certainly proved that she was a true friend, since as she said, "Mary Ellen and I always felt that we were friends, whether we were hanging out together or not. We were still there for each other as friends whenever we needed to be." Danielle had Mary Ellen's best interests at heart as she insisted that Mary Ellen should and could carry her own books and could do for herself. Danielle indicated, "It was very frustrating for me to see everyone pampering her because it was my feeling that I wanted her to be back to her independent self like she had been, so we could get back to going places and doing things." Danielle added: "Lots of us used to carry her books, but one day I got sick of this and told her, 'I'm going to carry your crutch instead of your books.'" Again Danielle felt it was time that Mary Ellen moved on and worked with one crutch so she could hurry up and progress to using just a cane. Danielle admits, "I know it was upsetting to her, my reaction about the crutches, and I'm sure she thought I was letting her down. But it did help her in the long run, and very soon she adapted to the cane."

Danielle and Mary Ellen found themselves in many a predicament because of Danielle's driving. One night, as Danielle chauffeured Mary Ellen, Katherine, and Lisa Gulotta home from catechism, trying to be cautious since the roads were snowy, they slid off the road into an embankment. They decided that Mary Ellen should assume the driver's seat as the three girls tried to push the car back on the road. They suddenly realized that with the clutch, brake, and gas pedal and only one leg, Mary Ellen couldn't possibly do the job.

Another experience with Danielle's car occurred when they came home very late one evening from babysitting and ran out of gas near the American Legion Hall in Sheffield, about two miles from Danielle's house. Mary Ellen announced, "We'll walk to your house."

Danielle told her, "That's not such a good idea. It's 2 o'clock in the morning!" As they sat and pondered their next move, a young man they recognized as "Red Dog"—nicknamed so because of a huge crop of bright red hair—stopped by and offered assistance.

Danielle later reported, "My father wasn't too happy that a person named 'Red Dog' had driven us home."

Danielle and Mary Ellen shared so many happy times during their high school days that it was inevitable that they remained very close friends as they went their separate ways; always calling and writing, keeping in touch. Danielle and Mary Ellen talked about the fun times and left the serious discussions for others. Danielle remembers, "I guess we always knew that our time together was too short and that we had to have fun in the short time we would have each other. We never discussed the seriousness of her illness."

During the assembly, Bob Krol, Mount Everett's guidance counselor and the girls' softball coach, called me into his offce and gave me a check—money donated by the Mount Everett family of teachers, staff, and school committee members. My first reaction was, "I can't take this."

Bob replied, "This gift comes from everyone who is experiencing your pain and sorrow, from all of us who want to and who have a right to help."

Never before had we had to receive. Until now, we had been so very fortunate that we usually found ourselves giving rather than being in a position of receiving. I took the check and told Bob, "This will start our Boston Fund to help defray the cost of the many, many trips back and forth to the hospital."

During this time of distress, we found it difficult at first to accept readily the outpouring of gifts, some monetary. Everyone was so genuinely concerned that we realized our friends in the community were reaching out to us, and so we learned to accept graciously and gladly all expressions of love and friendship. How lucky we were during those years of struggle to have such loyal and caring friends who made our battle that much easier. Sue Kinsley's spaghetti dinners and her offer to "sit" with Mary Ellen if she were too ill to go to school, like Sabrina Chapin's offers to "sit," were so appreciated. There were many others who played important parts in our struggle and who will be mentioned as Mary Ellen's story unfolds.

10

ॐ

ON DECEMBER 24 MARY ELLEN RECEIVED A LETTER FROM Channing Murdock, the owner of Butternut Basin, the ski area where she and Katherine had spent so many fun weekends. Channing wrote:

Dear Mary Ellen,
Merry Christmas! I was so glad to see you up and around here at Butternut the other day after such a trying experience. Your spirit is unbelievable and with such a positive outlook, I feel certain that you will overcome your difficulties and continue to experience the joys of life which you have until now.

I have found that you have already purchased a season pass, and enclose a check to reimburse you for the cost of this pass. As I mentioned to you, I want you to ski with us as my guest this winter, so if you haven't picked up your pass already, do so and enjoy it.

Einar [director of the ski school] is most anxious to work with you using the outriggers, and I'm sure you will find it a new and exciting challenge.

While in the hospital, Mary Ellen received a letter from a skiing buddy, John Street, who lived in New Canaan, Connecticut, and who skied with his family at Butternut on weekends and school vacations. John's letter also exemplifies the true essence of friendship:

Dear Mel,
At the end of last year, actually the end of last winter, I was really getting depressed. I was hard-pressed to get good grades, as I was taking two college courses along with several honors courses. Because of school work, I never got to bed before 1 a.m. and I had to get up four days a week for morning diving practice at 4:45. I split wood for our house and dove three hours each day. With all this, I didn't have any time for friends at home. I don't know how much of this I showed, but you responded. Even if you didn't realize it, you were the best friend I had. You always laughed and talked with me and rode up the lift with me when I was

about to go single. You were the one friend that I was able to count on, and you helped me stay sane for the rest of the season. Thank you so much, friend.

I know that you are going to be going through a lot rougher times than I ever went through, but I want you to know that I'm ready to help as much as I can. Don't let yourself get down. You've got a line of friends waiting to help you out. Friends can be the most valuable thing you'll have all of your life, and we'll always be ready to help you when you need it. Thank you for being such a friend to me, Mel. I'll always be here if you need me.

Each day Mary Ellen received new encouragement from all of her friends. She knew she would have staunch supporters from Day One. This support made her battle, and ours, easier. So as we fought during these next few years, we met many who fought with us, who became unforgettable allies.

11
❦

ON DECEMBER 21, JIM JR., MARY ELLEN, KATHERINE, JIMMY, AND I returned to Boston. Our first appointment was at the Jimmy Fund Pediatric Clinic. Here we again met Dr. Alan Goorin and Dr. Eva Guinan, who would become Mary Ellen's oncologist. Dr. Guinan, as beautiful a person inside as outside—petite, with dark hair and a flawless complexion—struck us with her youthful appearance. (Dr. Guinan had graduated from Harvard Medical School and had completed her residency in pediatrics at Children's Hospital. At the present time, Dr. Guinan is on the staff of the Dana-Farber as well as Children's Hospital.) In the five and a half years that Mary Ellen was her patient, she was always there for Mary Ellen and for us.

The first order of the day was to tell the doctors that Mary Ellen had decided against the randomization and would indeed become

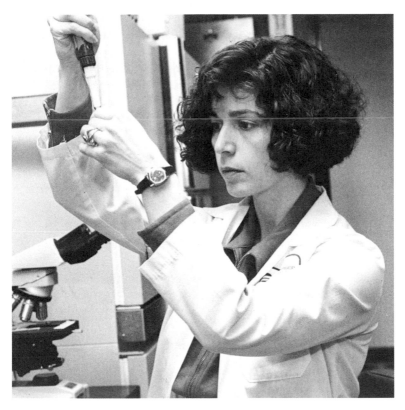

Dr. Eva Guinan

a candidate for the chemotherapy protocol. They then discussed the procedures and gave us material to read and sign, along with a schedule of chemo protocol. They emphasized that Mary Ellen should become familiar with all the drugs she would ultimately receive, knowing how to pronounce them and knowing all their side effects. Our vocabulary began to include this new terminology, so that the terms and names of drugs eventually became second nature. We were especially told of all the possible side effects; the major ones being extreme nausea, hair loss, and weight loss.

After the discussion with Dr. Guinan and Dr. Goorin, we made the first appointment for the chemo treatment on December 28.

Mary Ellen and I would go to Boston, and I'd stay with the Rinkles for the duration of the treatment. We were still on Christmas vacation, so school was no problem.

The protocol Mary Ellen would undergo was designed to combat the cancer cells, to kill them, if possible, so that they would not metastasize (spread) to the lungs. Knowing all of the side effects, we wondered if Mary Ellen would be able to cope with them while traveling back and forth to Boston, going to school, and trying to maintain her everyday routine. No one can comprehend the whole chemo protocol unless it is experienced. Through Mary Ellen we experienced this ordeal—watching her lose weight; lose hair; become nauseous, violently at times; and experience painful mouth sores.

After our meeting with the doctors, we went to the hospital brace shop, where she received her temporary prosthesis. Sal LaBella was on hand to help her get used to her new limb. Because we had continued to wrap her stump carefully, as Shelley had directed, Mary Ellen did not have too difficult a time putting on her "leg." As Sal directed, Mary Ellen first put on a heavy "sock" and then lowered her limb into the socket. A Salesian Belt (a belt two inches wide), attached to the prosthesis was worn around the waist, thus ensuring the leg's adhesion. With this temporary arrangement, Mary Ellen started out using crutches for balance and mobility, and to decrease the weight bearing on the not-fully-healed scarring. This healing would be slowed down later by the chemo. After a while, she was able to resort to just one crutch. On this monumental day, however, she used the two crutches. As soon as the prosthesis was on and Sal had checked the fit, he determined that after a visit with Shelley, who would give more instructions on wearing the leg, and a week's practice at home, we would probably need another appointment for a follow-up. This we made for the 28th, when Mary Ellen would be confined to the hospital for the first chemo treatment. Any changes to be made to the prosthesis could be done then.

We had had a full day and were glad now to return home to enjoy the holidays. During the next few days, we received many letters and cards wishing Mary Ellen well as she and we embarked on this next phase of combatting the disease. A good friend, Iona Brigham, who had had a mastectomy performed a few years before, visited and talked about her experiences with chemo. She had received some of the same drugs Mary Ellen would experience. Iona noted, "I was one of the lucky ones not to lose my hair. Perhaps you'll have the same luck." Iona's visit helped, since she gave Mary Ellen an idea about the treatments. We hoped Mary Ellen would be as lucky as Iona.

Part 2

1

❧

ON DECEMBER 28, MARY ELLEN AND I DROVE TO THE JIMMY Fund Clinic for the start of the first treatment, Cytoxan. As soon as we arrived, her height, weight, and blood pressure were recorded since these statistics were vital in determining the dosage of the drug. After this, we went downstairs for an X-ray, an important procedure because it checked the condition of the lungs and noted if there were any metastases. Each and every visit made to the Clinic for the next five and a half years began in the same manner. After we checked in with Dr. Guinan, the IV nurse, usually Mary Foley, put in the IV and then, with Mary Ellen attached to the IV, we used a wheelchair and a volunteer to take us to Children's. The trip could be made without going outside, using passageways and elevators.

We were soon on our way to Children's, to Division 36, where the chemo would be administered. From this very first day, we learned to carry an emesis basin or, as we so aptly called, a "spit-up pan." This became part of our traveling equipment, along with a towel and a pillow. Mary Ellen became nauseous immediately, now succumbing to her nerves, later vomiting because of the drugs. Nothing seemed to help as she continued to vomit for the duration of the treatment.

As soon as we arrived on the floor, the nurses settled Mary Ellen into her bed. Over the years, she probably inhabited every bed in every room on Division 36. The nurses, especially Ellen Z were always available to make her comfortable. Usually the chemo began in the late afternoon. Each of the six drugs was administered in a slightly different manner, but for the most part Mary Ellen was confined to a bed or wheelchair during the treatment time. This first time, I stayed each day with her and helped to take care of her, emptying the "spit-up pan" and the bedpan. Anything I could do for her I did. Much later on in our struggle, I remarked to the nurses, "By now I think I have at least earned a LPN degree."

Each time we went to Boston, thirteen months in all, Mary Ellen stayed a minimum of three days and a maximum of seven. As soon as we got into the car at home, she became nauseous. Her mood changed as she became quiet and withdrawn. This behavior was understandable, since she knew there would be IV's, blood tests, poking and prodding, along with the nausea while she was confined to bed. The nausea usually continued through the treatment until she left the hospital and we started for home. She ate little, drinking only apple juice or iced tea.

During these months of chemo, many of our friends came to our assistance and drove us to and from Boston, 136 miles each way. These friends—Betsy Smith, Holly Coon, Chris Chapin, the Saderas, Maureen Seward, Scott Cary, Cathy Archey, John Peron, Kim Emprimo, Ann Makuc, Sue Kinsley—saved us a great deal of emotional distress, not to mention the wear and tear on our car. We left the driving to them and our only concern then became Mary Ellen's well-being.

Each trip we made (there were twenty-two treatments) followed the same plan. We'd leave Sheffield about 7 a.m., planning to arrive at the Jimmy Fund Clinic about 10. After Mary Ellen was admitted and settled in her bed, usually about 2 p.m., we'd make the return trip. If it were a school vacation I'd stay, but most of the time we'd return home. If Mary Ellen had wanted us to stay, we would have; but she knew Jimmy and I had our jobs to do and understood it was almost impossible for us to stay through each treatment. During these hospital stays she slept a great deal, and therefore she said, "What will you do all week, just sit here and look at me?" This was Mary Ellen's way of telling us she could really handle the treatments without us. Sometimes I felt sad leaving her, especially as she lay in bed waiting for the treatment to begin and using the "spit-up pan" periodically. I also knew that by being there, there were ways I could help the nurses to do little things for her. Our jobs, however, were necessary and even though our respective employers were understanding, we felt we had to return to work.

The nurses were marvelous, giving us such peace of mind that we didn't worry. Friends and relatives in Boston—the Rinkles,

Margaret Ball, Marie Driscoll, and Frances Benedict—volunteered to look in on her. We telephoned several times each day. Of course, the nurses would have called immediately if there were a problem. All in all, we supported Mary Ellen even when we were at home and she was in Boston. A note from Joan Widell of the physical therapy department at Children's filled us with pride as she talked about our part in Mary Ellen's struggle. Joan wrote.

Dear Mr. and Mrs. Welch,
I wanted you to know how much I've always admired the ways in which you were able to support Mary Ellen in her battle with cancer. There are few parents who can be so open about their anger at the disease (how loved she must have felt), hold their daughter's hand through difficult surgeries and chemotherapy, and still be able to let her grow and live her short life to the fullest. No wonder Mary Ellen was such a special person—she was part of you. I'll always treasure my memories of Mary Ellen and her wonderful parents.

2
❦

USUALLY OUR TRIPS WERE UNEVENTFUL. HOWEVER, I VIVIDLY remember one trip in January. Maureen Seward and Jim Jr. were with Mary Ellen and me. We had had several inches of snow the day before and, as we left the turnpike to take Route 128, we noticed the snow had blown against the exit signs, covering the numbers. Being novices when it came to making the trip, we were still a bit unsure of the Route 9 exit. We finally agreed upon the exit, left 128, and traveled along Route 9 toward the hospital. The traffic moved quite slowly because of the snow, until it came to a complete standstill. This particular treatment was to be Methotrexate, and all of Mary Ellen's vital information had to be delivered to the hospital by noon so the pharmacy would have time to prepare the dosage. The treatment would begin in the late afternoon;

otherwise, if we were late with the vital statistics, treatment would begin the following day, thereby lengthening her stay in the hospital. With all of these thoughts going through our heads, we anxiously observed the slowdown as we moved inch by inch. An hour had passed and we had gone only one-half-mile.

Being unfamiliar with the area, we hadn't yet learned the side roads and shortcuts. As we approached a traffic light, we noticed a few cars turning left. Then I spotted a hospital laundry truck and said to Maureen, "Follow the truck! He must be going to the hospital."

Maureen turned off Route 9 and we followed the truck: up and down, in and out some winding residential streets. As luck would have it, in a few minutes we found ourselves in Brookline Village, about five minutes from the Farber. Had we not followed the truck, who knows how long we would have been waiting. We certainly were lucky, with all the hospitals in Boston, to have found a truck heading toward our hospital.

We never considered the trips to Boston to be out of the question. Several times neighbors and acquaintances would ask if there were hospitals and doctors closer. However, after our initial trip to Children's, we came to the conclusion that we were indeed fortunate that Dr. Hajek and Dr. Gallup had sent us there. The staffs at all of the hospitals—Dana-Farber, Children's, and the Brigham—were the best. We met people from far-away countries as well as from many states who had traveled to Children's because of its outstanding reputation. When we were first introduced to the Jimmy Fund staff, we were also very grateful that we had the best going for us. If anyone could help us fight our battle, these professionals certainly could. The constant discussions and conferences carried on, especially those directed by Dr. Eva Guinan, filled us with hope. Not one avenue was left unexplored, as Dr. Guinan consulted many other physicians during Mary Ellen's treatments. We are thankful for all their expertise and know that Mary Ellen's life was prolonged because of the dedication of these knowledgeable doctors who were associated with her case. In June, 1988, after Mary Ellen's death, Dr. Guinan said to us, "You are never to reproach yourselves with 'what ifs.' Mary Ellen knew that you and we did everything humanly possible for her."

We know this to be true. We didn't win the war, but we surely put up a gallant fight.

3

WHEN JIMMY, KATHERINE, JIM JR, AND I VISITED DR. GUINAN after Mary Ellen's death, we said in all honesty, "No matter what each visit brought—good news or bad—you always gave us hope to pursue all possibilities. You had the ability to take us from the depths of an unpleasant diagnosis so that upon leaving your office we felt a ray of hope that all was not lost." Dr. Guinan helped us battle the disease every step of the way. Mary Ellen looked upon her not only as her doctor but also as her friend and confidant.

Dr. Guinan commented on some of the aspects of Mary Ellen's struggle by saying, "All we understand is how much of this struggle is not singular but how much of it is really process, not just process for the patient, but for the family, too. It's process for the doctor and for the nurses, especially with someone her age. She was at an age where she really had a personality, a being, an age. And to see how this person grew and changed and developed..."

I interjected, "I could see how she grew. At first she hated Boston and the hospital. She hated the whole chemotherapy thing. We couldn't blame her. Then she changed, I think, after the first long protocol was completed and she spent a day with Shelley observing the physical therapy program. At first, she exhibited an interest in a career in physical therapy but decided against such a difficult program because of her limitations in the math and science fields. She did think, however, that maybe she could help young people by taking up a career in rehabilitation." (This she did when she majored in Pediatric Rehabilitation at Springfield College.)

Dr. Guinan continued talking about the process, saying, "I think a patient like Mary Ellen is old enough and verbal enough to really interact with people. Here was a bilateral interaction. But, as you have said, the family interacted with the community and them with you. Sometimes from the beginning you don't want people in your life. You just want to deal with it and have it over. It's not one of those things that gets over with quickly. And I think one of the things you see here is that people either really try to keep themselves isolated, which is pretty generally unsuccessful for them as a coping strategy, or really do sort of end up finding a way to interact with their family, friends, support network, ministers—whatever is helpful for them. Some people are luckier than others. Mary Ellen had some wonderful friends, which is likely a testament to her in terms of the friends she attracted."

Dr. Guinan concluded, "I can't think of anything you could have done differently. It would have been really terrific if this all hadn't happened, but I can't think of anything that we could have done, either, or that anyone could have done that would have made it any easier."

It is my firm belief that we can't lose sight of the Divine Plan which God has ordained, that we are on this earth for a reason, and it is not up to us to question how long our term on earth shall be. Mary Ellen in her twenty-two years lived life to its fullest and contributed selflessly of her time and energy to others. She had a very positive effect upon those with whom she came in contact. And so, as Dr. Guinan said, "It would have been great if this hadn't happened." But it did happen, and we all coped with the illness to the best of our ability. Mary Ellen particularly was the star in her own story. By her acceptance, she took a very difficult situation and turned it into a positive experience.

4

WE NOW HAD ONE CHEMO TREATMENT DOWN WITH TWENTY-ONE more to go. The chart of treatments hung on the refrigerator, and as each one ended, we checked it off. With this first treatment we worried about hair loss, since everyone told Mary Ellen to expect it. On the wall of the Jimmy Fund Clinic is a poster depicting Charlie Brown with the words "Bald is beautiful." This poster acts as a constant reminder of this major side effect.

About two or three weeks after her first treatment, as Mary Ellen finished showering, she yelled, "Come quick!"

Not knowing what had happened, I ran to the bathroom, and there on the floor were clumps of her beautiful long, dark blond hair. Mary Ellen sobbed as we took a towel and picked up the hair from the floor. This was one of the very few times that Mary Ellen really cried, but seeing her beautiful hair on the floor was too devastating. We hadn't investigated wigs, but as she began to lose her hair, we realized the need for one. A friend at Mount Everett told me of a hairdresser in Pittsfield who specialized in wigs. We made an appointment and planned to order one.

On a cold, windy Saturday morning, Jim Jr. drove Mary Ellen and me to Pittsfield to meet with the hairdresser. She had just a few little strands of hair left, so determining the exact color by looking at a small sample was difficult. We finally chose a color and style and ordered the wig. In the meantime, Mary Ellen seemed content wearing a bandanna; in fact, she really wasn't too keen on a wig and just seemed to be going along with what her father and I felt was best.

A week later the wig arrived, and we returned for a fitting and a trim. There she was with hair again. She wore the wig home, and much to our dismay, took it off immediately, covering her head with one of her favorite bandannas. One of Mary Ellen's strongest character traits was her stubborness, and this was obvious on the wig subject. I believe she wore this wig only three times: at a lunch with the Kennedys that winter, at her Confirmation in May 1983, and at the Junior-Senior prom in late May 1983. I think the reason she felt uncomfortable wearing it was that the wig was not Mary Ellen; it was fake, and Mary Ellen definitely did not indulge in things that were fake. She'd rather go without hair, wearing her bandanna.

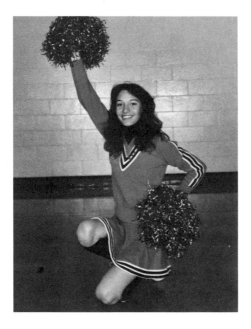

Denise

Denise Sadera, a Mount Everett classmate, tells of two incidents regarding Mary Ellen's loss of hair. One related to Luke Moulton and his struggle with cancer. Luke, the young son of a neighbor, had lost his beautiful red hair at first but it began to grow back. Mary Ellen told Denise, "Maybe my hair will grow back like Luke's, a beautiful red! And when it does, we'll have a bandanna burning!"

Another incident occurred before a basketball game at Mount Everett. Denise, a cheerleader, and Mary Ellen were standing in the foyer as Denise checked her hair, using the big glass window of the office for a mirror. The opposing team's cheerleaders were doing the same farther on down the hall, but they were also staring at Mary Ellen. She had become accustomed to people staring at her cane and her bandanna, often commenting, "I wonder what they're thinking?" This time Mary Ellen, always ready to take advantage of a situation, asked Denise, "Let me borrow your comb." She then proceeded to comb her bandanna as she gazed at her image in the window, inquiring, "Is my part straight? How does my hair look?" The other cheerleaders, embarrassed by their inquisitiveness, hastened into the gym.

5
❦

AS THE TREATMENTS PROGRESSED, IF WE NEEDED A PLACE TO stay, we could still make use of the Rinkles' apartment in Newton. In February, 1983, as we drove in from Newton one Sunday morning, a snowstorm made the Boston streets slippery. We usually went to Mass at St. Aidan's in Brookline, but with the roads so slippery, we were convinced we'd never make the 8 o'clock service. Driving along Commonwealth Avenue, we noticed people going into St. Ignatius Church at Boston College and decided to go to Mass there. As we went up the aisle for communion, a person behind Jimmy put her hand on his arm. He turned and saw his cousin, Margaret Ball. After Mass, we returned to Margaret's apartment and told her about Mary Ellen. Margaret maintained her family home in Great Barrington but also lived in Boston, where she worked as a biochemist at The Brigham and Women's Hospital.

Since Jimmy and Margaret did not see one another very often, she didn't know about Mary Ellen's illness. After breakfast, as we unfolded our story, Margaret told us that we were to consider her apartment our home. She had a key made for us and told the neighbors about us, so they, too, made us feel welcome. Her apartment was on the T line (Massachusetts Transit) so we could easily leave our car in the parking area and take the transit car to the hospital. Had it not been snowing and had we been able to get to Mass in Brookline, who knows how long it would have been before we touched base with Margaret?

When we told Johanna and Roy Rinkle about "finding" Margaret, they were also delighted. They understood our staying with Margaret, but they still extended the invitation to use their place any time we needed a home. On that morning as we left Margaret's, the snow still fell as we drove down Commonwealth to the hospital to visit Mary Ellen before returning home. I just happened to glance out the car window and there, waiting for the T, was John Tuller from Great Barrington. We would have stopped, but the traffic and snow made it a bit difficult. What a coincidence! Two Great Barrington natives in one morning!

6
❦

EACH TIME WE WENT FOR A TREATMENT, WE SCHEDULED AN appointment with Shelley for a check on the prosthesis and for some physical therapy. Sometimes the prosthesis went to the brace shop for adjustments. These could be done while Mary Ellen was confined to bed. Shelley kept after Mary Ellen about exercising, since sometimes she became a bit lazy and put it off more than she should. Shelley emphasized the fact that exercise was vital to her well-being. The PT sessions with Shelley were not as effective as they should have been due to Mary Ellen's being nauseous. They had only a small portion of a session prior to the chemo. She usually arrived at her appointment with Shelley carrying the "spit-up pan." Because the emphasis of the PT was improvement of the gait, with the increased strength and flexibility to do so, Shelley decided that PT closer to home would be necessary. Jack

Lloyd, associated with Sharon Hospital in Sharon, Connecticut, agreed to work long distance with Shelley and directly with Mary Ellen two or three times a week. While working with Jack, Mary Ellen tossed aside the crutches when Jack one day presented her with a cane, the one she continued to use throughout her struggle. From then on, the crutches were used only when the prosthesis was off, primarily in the evening.

During the long protocol, Dr. Gallup came to our assistance regarding the blood tests. These were necessary to determine the time of each subsequent treatment and so were usually administered beginning on the tenth day after treatment had begun and continued until the results proved in order for the next treatment. Again we drove to Sharon Hospital for these tests. Dr. Gallup merely told the lab that anytime we needed a test done, they were to please comply with our request. This they did, again making this procedure routine. About two hours after each test, I would call the lab for the results and then telephone them to Dr. Guinan, who would then arrange the next treatment date. I became very proficient in recording these results. CBC (complete blood count); WBC (white blood count); hematocrit (a red blood cell component); hemoglobin (the iron-protein component in the red blood cells that carries oxygen to the tissue); polys, lymphs, monos, and basos (these are kinds of white blood cells); and platelets (a main component of the blood that forms clots that seal up injured areas to prevent hemorrhage) became a part of our everyday working vocabulary.

As Mary Ellen proceeded with her life, we seemed to have all bases covered. She went along "doing her thing" as before, with skiing the only activity she actively missed. However, visits to Butternut were frequent, with promises of "next year." While undergoing the chemo treatments, it was not considered advisable for her to ski. Besides facing loss of weight due to nausea, the healing process of her stump was slowed down because of the drugs.

During the trips back and forth to Boston, Mary Ellen also continued her studies at Mount Everett. The administration and teachers realized she would have difficulty keeping up with all of her courses, so they were helpful by giving her extensions, particularly in history and English. Not being a math wizard (and not having the genes to be one), Mary Ellen found geometry too difficult and dropped the class, but otherwise her program remained intact.

It's ironic that cancer struck at this time. One day, previous to the amputation, Mary Ellen admitted, "I'm really into school this year." Her first report card, about two weeks before the diagnosis, was a terrific one. She continued, "I'm into studying and liking school now. In the ninth grade I didn't like myself, and tenth grade was my year of rebellion."

We never realized she had felt this way. We thought we knew our kids, and I, especially, being a teacher, always seemed to pinpoint these situations in other children. Mary Ellen had put on some weight, and even with soccer, field hockey, softball, skiing, and swimming, she was still a little "chunky." She declared, "I was really fat."

Her sister was quite thin, and as Mary Ellen's friend Lisa Gulotta said, "Mary Ellen was jealous of Katherine's being so thin."

School became important to Mary Ellen. Not only the academics, but all of the other activities became a vital part of her life. She was a true Eagle fan, yelling the teams on to victory whether she played on the team or rooted from the sidelines. After the amputation, she continued to be Mount Everett's biggest fan. She struggled with treatments, blood tests, trips to Boston, nausea—everything that went with the illness. She worked hard at her classes and passed. How easy it would have been to have thrown in the towel and to sit back, letting school slide. Had she done that, perhaps no one would have blamed her. However, none of us let that alternative cross our minds. Rather, she picked up where she had left off before the diagnosis and worked as hard as she could. She had set as her goal a college education, and we supported her all the way.

Throughout her struggle, therefore, she realized the importance of continuing her education and of doing well. Even during the last few months before her death, when the cancer seemed to have the upper hand and appeared to be winning the battle, she worried about her classes. While at Springfield College in April 1988, she had to drop two or three courses. She worried, "I'll never finish." We told her if it took six years to complete her college degree who would care? We supported her desire to remain at school even though going to classes proved more and more trying.

7

IN FEBRUARY 1983, CHANNING MURDOCK ARRANGED A LUNCH for all of us to meet Ted Kennedy Jr., who had also lost his leg to bone cancer; his mother, Joan; and his younger brother, Patrick. The Kennedys visited Butternut during the school vacation. Mary Ellen, having been on chemo for a month and a half at this point, had lost all of her hair. Because of this special event, Jimmy and I felt the wig was in order. It was our pleasure to meet the Kennedys, and in discussing the disease, Joan Kennedy stated, "You know, Mary Ellen will lose her hair."

I answered, looking at Mary Ellen and grinning, "She already has."

We didn't think the wig was so terrible, but the only reason Mary Ellen wore it on this day was to appease Jimmy and me. If she had had her way, she would have chosen a bandanna.

Bandannas were her style. She wore them most of the time, even to bed. We would ask her, "Why the bandanna to bed?"

She'd come back with, "I don't want my head to get cold."

She had different colored bandannas to match all of her sweaters. Since she experienced complete hair loss three different times during her struggle, bandannas became an important part of her wardrobe. Once a new outfit called for a black bandanna. Until she found the right one, she wouldn't wear the outfit. During a time when her hair had grown back, she and Amy, her roommate at Springfield, decorated the heating pipe in their dorm room with bandannas. Green, yellow, blue, red, pink—bandannas of every conceivable color were wrapped from floor to ceiling. Another time, a sign went up on the door, "Bandannas for Sale—fifty cents."

Skiing, her favorite of all sports, had to be put on hold for the 1983 season since the chemo was taking its toll. This was a bitter pill because all of her friends took off on Saturdays and Sundays for Butternut. She and Katherine were so into the sport that during the previous August we had taken advantage of the sales and had gone to Pittsfield to buy new jackets and coordinating hats. As we drove home in 90° weather, with the windows rolled down, Mary Ellen and Katherine sported their new ski jackets and waved at all as we drove by. Skiing was on their minds almost all year long!

About two weeks after the amputation, we went to Butternut to talk with Einar Aas, the ski school director, about outriggers. We wanted to alert Einar to be ready for Mary Ellen the following season. He assured us he would get the necessary equipment and have everything ready. At this time Mary Ellen really didn't feel up to skiing but was rather content to go to Butternut to sit in the sun on the deck, to watch Katherine and others, and to just be there with her friends. Occasionally Jimmy, Mary Ellen, and I arrived at noon to meet our friends from Larchmont, Helga and Vic Pisani and their four sons. We sat in the sun, eating sandwiches and drinking a glass of wine as Mark, Jason, Craig, and Keith Pisani and Katherine skied. We spent many a pleasant afternoon while Mary Ellen looked forward to 1984, the completion of chemo and joining the others on the slopes.

8
❦

ON MARCH 17, MARY ELLEN RECEIVED A NEW TEMPORARY PROS-
thesis, which fit much better than the original one since her stump
had become stronger. On March 21, four days before her seven-
teenth birthday, she was to undergo another treatment with
Methotrexate. She dreaded this drug because it had a terrible side
effect—mouth sores—and also because blood tests taken after the
five- or six-day ordeal had to show the Methotrexate level down to
.01 before she could be discharged. The primary reason for this
was to avoid dehydration if severe vomiting occurred. This time
the nurses gave a little surprise birthday party, with a resident, Dr.
Peter Havens, leading the birthday parade. Dr. Havens, always
thinking of Mary Ellen, asked the lab to do several blood tests
during the last day of the rescue drug Leucovorin (used to lower
the Methotrexate level and to clear the kidneys). He knew how
badly Mary Ellen wanted to get out of the hospital. Finally, the
tests showed a good level and we were quickly on our way home.
The following week, we celebrated Mary Ellen's birthday with a
little party at home. Mary Ellen couldn't eat but had to be content
just to drink, since the awful mouth sores had materialized. With
the nurses' remedy of mouthwash, water, and peroxide available,
she managed to keep the sores under control and finally get rid of
them. Luckily, she experienced the sores only once more during
the protocol.

9

💙

MARCH AND APRIL PASSED WITH SOFTBALL PRACTICE KEEPING Katherine and Mary Ellen busy. Mary Ellen had pitched for the team and planned to do so again, but while she was wearing the temporary prosthesis, sports had to wait. For now, she was content to be the manager and the team's biggest supporter. Bob Krol, the softball coach, remembers this season immediately following the amputation: "Before Mel's operation, I was a coach in the enviable position of having two girls named Welch developing as fast-pitch windmill-style softball pitchers. Both Katherine and Mel worked very hard to develop their skills. But when Mel lost her leg, I admit I gave up on her and concentrated on her sister, Katherine. In that first season back, in an attempt to find a place for Mel, I assigned her as third base coach. Picture Mel standing out there at third, at first on crutches and later with a cane, screaming instructions to her teammates. That role was short-lived as the Umpires Association voted not to allow her to stand there 'for her own safety.' I guess they gave up on her, too." Mary Ellen remained the staunch fan from the bench just waiting until the next year.

With May came the Junior-Senior prom. Marcia Brolli and I were junior class advisors, responsible for overseeing the prom details. This year it was to be held at Butternut Basin, thanks to the generosity of Channing Murdock. We all worked long and hard on the decorations, and the result of our labors was the transformation of the lower lodge into a beautiful pink and white fairyland. Mary Ellen invited Keith Pisani. Katherine also went to the prom as did Jimmy and I. This was the third time Mary Ellen wore her wig. We told her that with a floor-length white lace dress, a bandanna just would not be a good fashion statement. We decorated her crutches with pink ribbons and flowers. She and Katherine were heard to remark that it was almost a family affair, since the four of us attended. Jimmy, much to their dismay, came armed with his camera. It was a fun evening, even though the girls said they were "embarrassed" by their father's photography.

In June Mary Ellen completed her junior year at Mount Everett and planned to work during the summer on an American history term paper and a few history chapters for her teacher, Jim Herlihy. During the school year, to make things easier for her, Jim Jr. read the history chapters and wrote out the answers to the questions. Mary Ellen told Mr. Herlihy, with her fingers crossed, "I did the work, but I had to dictate the answers to the questions because of the IV in my right hand."

The history term paper remained the last history assignment to be done. One morning I made the announcement, "We are going to begin this paper now, and we are not going to get up from the table until it's done." By 5 o'clock that afternoon, Mary Ellen had finished the paper, entitled "The Effects of the Depression on Farmers, the Unemployed, and Children."

Mary Ellen also had a few assignments in English to complete, the last one being a term paper. Scott Cary, her English teacher, came to the house a few times to help her. She planned to write the paper on osteogenic sarcoma. Before she could begin, however, she had to find the sources and material to develop a well-planned paper. Where else to find the material than from those involved in her treatment? Dr. Kramer was the resident doctor as she planned the paper. He agreed to help. One day as Mary Ellen went through the usual admission process before a treatment, Dr. Kramer and I went to the library in Children's where he took the time to photocopy material and sources. Peggy, one of the nurses at the Jimmy Fund Clinic, gave Mary Ellen a few books that also were valuable sources. This was just another incident illustrating the caring and concern that all of her doctors and nurses exhibited. Mary Ellen received an A on her paper. By August, she had completed all of her assignments and officially became a senior.

Besides completing all of her schoolwork, Mary Ellen also took driving lessons, passed the test, and earned her license. We had a left-foot gas pedal installed so she could use the car. The license really made her feel more independent, for she could now go places with friends and not have to rely on someone to drive her.

10

Ꮗ

SWIMMING AT MY FATHER'S POOL IN HILLSDALE, JUST OVER the New York border, along with picnics with family and friends helped to make the summer a fun one—as much as it could be fun with the treatments still continuing. Mary Ellen loved to swim and to "catch the rays." The latter was a no-no during the treatments, since sun and chemo don't go hand-in-hand, but she did cheat a bit when it came to getting a tan. Mary Ellen took her lack of leg in stride, thereby putting others at ease. Occasionally there would be a guest at the pool who had a difficult time dealing with her loss, but eventually Mary Ellen's attitude took over. Sometimes Aunt Rita, the only one of the senior citizens (the elderly guests— Aunt Rita, Aunt Ruth, Aunt Marian, and Uncle Frank) who swam, would say how sad she felt, seeing Mary Ellen. But she, too, became accustomed to the loss of the limb. Before the end of that first summer, no one seemed to be bothered as they took the turn of events in stride. However, Mary Ellen refrained from swimming at the pools of friends, especially at parties with many guests. When we went to the beach at the Cape or New Hampshire, she did go swimming, and tossed aside any curious glances.

We all looked forward to the annual July Fourth picnic in Hillsdale, when family and friends came together for a celebration with swimming, games, and lots of food. Grandpa's favorite expression as we all arrived and the grandchildren and children ran to the pool was, "Don't forget to bring the children." This particular summer, my brother Joseph brought a huge beribboned box, which occupied a prominent place on the patio. This intriguing red, white, and blue box was the subject of a guessing game. We all took turns. No one except Aunt Rita, who we think cheated, could figure out the contents. When the box was opened, there were fifty ice cream cones, all different flavors, packed in dry ice. We ate cones during the rest of the week as we stored the leftovers in the freezer.

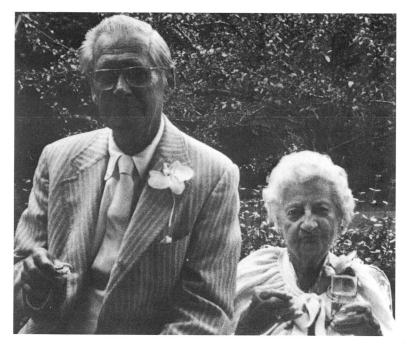

Grandpa and Nanny

The house in Hillsdale, where Nanny and Grandpa spent a few months of the year, became a fun place for the kids. Grandpa was truly concerned about Mary Ellen, and never a day went by that he did not ask about her. She and Grandpa had a special relationship, and as the years went by and Mary Ellen continued her fight, he was always there to give moral support. After each visit to Boston, he would call to ask the results. Sometimes, when the news wasn't good, I'd hate to tell him. He and all of the "senior citizens" prayed for us and gave us a great deal of moral support. Grandpa kept a supply of $50 bills on hand, and each time Mary Ellen visited, he would press a folded bill into her hand. Katherine wore a long face when her sister showed her her newfound wealth. Often, however, Mary Ellen treated Katherine to lunch or to the movies with Grandpa's gift. Mary Ellen dearly loved her Grandpa, whom she affectionately called "Pops."

Before we returned to school in September, the girls and I

planned a short stay in Rye Beach, New Hampshire, renting a cottage that belonged to Jimmy's cousin's sister, Betty McKenna. Since the cottage had sleeping arrangements for five, each of the girls invited a friend. Mary Ellen, Danielle, Katherine, Jennifer Kinsley, and I spent a few great days again sunning ourselves, swimming, and just relaxing before school began. The stay in Rye Beach proved a welcome respite from the Boston trips.

11

IN SEPTEMBER, JIM JR. RESUMED HIS CLASSES AT THE STATE University of New York at Cobleskill, having been on a leave for three semesters. His being at home, even though he took classes at Berkshire Community College and worked at the Red Lion Inn in Stockbridge, had proved to be a great help whenever we needed someone to assist in the drive to Boston or just to help out. Katherine returned to Mount Everett as a junior and Mary Ellen entered her senior year. She took five subjects: English, Spanish, French, history, and geometry. She would again try to succeed with the math. In September, since she couldn't play soccer, Mary Ellen decided to be part of the team as the manager. We started out then with excitement, since this was the year of graduation.

At the start of the soccer season, Bob Krol introduced the team to Kelly Milan, a Great Barrington native and an outstanding soccer player at the University of Massachusetts who had been hired as a physical education aide. Besides her duties as an aide, Kelly would assist Bob with the team. A sincere friendship developed between Kelly and Mary Ellen, which spread to all of us. Throughout the battle with cancer, Kelly and her husband, Joe, gave us all kinds of support as we grew to know and love them as though they were truly family.

Mary Ellen attended almost all of the soccer games, but she

seemed to spend more time with Kelly's junior varsity team, walking up and down the sidelines with Kelly as she coached the girls. Kelly remembers when Mary Ellen fell during a practice. Someone had kicked the ball near where she was standing and Mary Ellen couldn't resist the urge to kick it back into play, when down she went. Kelly yelled, "Who kicked that ball there?" Kelly later reported, "I was really upset. Did it bother Mary Ellen? Of course not! She got up and continued on."

The relationship between Mary Ellen and Kelly that developed during these months was more than just a friendship. Mary Ellen thought of Kelly as an older sister. Kelly remembers the search for a Christmas tree, as she and Mary Ellen journeyed to Ashley Falls to a "cut your own" tree farm. They brought no saw, nor rope to tie the tree onto the car. Mary Ellen tripped over roots and terrain as they plowed their way through the rows of trees, trying to find the perfect one. As luck would have it, an acquaintance of Kelly's happened to be cutting his tree, so they inveigled him to help. He cut the tree they chose and gave them rope to tie it to the car. Kelly remembers vividly their driving up Route 7 and passing Jimmy on the way. He almost went off the road laughing, because they had tied the tree on backwards, and as they sped along, the branches were blowing uncontrollably. Jimmy followed them, and when they arrived at Kelly's, helped to untie the almost demolished tree, exclaiming, "Only you two could tie a tree backwards. You're lucky you have a tree and that the branches didn't all break off."

As the school year progressed, Kelly and Mary Ellen continued to support one another. Kelly, being new to the system, indicated Mary Ellen's concern for her well-being as she said:

Mary Ellen sort of took me under her wing. I was the newcomer and she the 'old pro.' I met so many kids through her. I felt as if she guided me my first year at Mount Everett. When I applied for the teaching position in the Phys. Ed. department, Mary Ellen became my champion. She attended the school committee meeting when my name was proposed, and as soon as the committee voted, she called me: 'Just want you to know you're a teacher.' She looked out for me and made my first year easier.

12

❦

IN OCTOBER THE SENIORS PREPARED FOR THEIR YEARBOOK
pictures. Mary Ellen, of course, still had no hair and we had not
had the foresight to arrange for a portrait before her hair loss.
Mary Ellen entertained the thought of not appearing in the yearbook. We all said, "Later on, as you glance through the yearbook
and you're not there, you're going to be really disappointed." We
all tried to convince her to have a picture with the wig. That
resulted in a flat "No way!" Then we suggested one wearing the
bandanna. We gradually wore down her defenses, and one day
Ken Langenbach arrived in the class with his camera. We prevailed
upon Mary Ellen to let Ken take her picture. She did so, and I'm
sure she was happy when she saw herself with the rest of her class
in the yearbook. We told her, "Years later, when your classmates
look at their yearbooks, they'll remember your struggle with
cancer."

The rest of the semester progressed routinely with Boston,
classes, dances, movies, and the hopes of skiing when the chemo
ended. This we targeted for February 1984. The protocol schedule
still hung on the refrigerator and showed that we were definitely
nearing the end. Mary Ellen also talked about the party she
expected when she finished the chemo. As she so aptly put it, "It'll
be the biggest and the bestest party."

After Christmas, Jimmy started to talk with Mary Ellen about
resuming skiing. He had spoken with Einar Aas, who with Jimmy
had purchased the outriggers. Into January, each weekend Jimmy
suggested the skiing, but Mary Ellen would find an excuse. I'm
sure she wanted to go in the worst way but was a bit scared. Finally,
one Saturday morning, Jimmy said, "Put on your ski clothes.
You're going today." Jimmy had become quite overprotective of
Mary Ellen, and was very solicitous of her well-being (a characteristic which at times annoyed Mary Ellen). He knew, however,
that she had to get back into the skiing atmosphere to be happy

and that we had to perhaps be forceful when it came to the initial "plunge." Therefore, Jimmy made arrangements with Einar to have an instructor show her the workings of the outriggers. Off they went, Mary Ellen with the ski hat pulled down over the bandanna. After reaching the bunny slope and going up in the chair, she and the instructor started down the slope. At the bottom about twenty of Mary Ellen's skiing buddies had gathered—watching and waiting anxiously for her to make her first run. As she came down the slope, using the outriggers, the old joy of skiing returned once more. How the kids all cheered as she made her first run! Another "Standing O" was hers. From that time on, no more bunny slope, but rather to the top of Free Wheeler and Lucifer's and the other more difficult slopes. A wipe-out, which was rare, just meant getting back up and continuing on her way with a big grin and a wave.

13
❦

THE LAST TREATMENT OCCURRED IN JANUARY. HOLLY COON drove us to Boston this time. As the doctors checked Mary Ellen, particularly her mouth since they thought she might have the beginnings of sores, Holly and I waited. All of a sudden, Mary Ellen came running out of the office, laughing and crying at the same time. "I'm done," she yelled to us. "I don't need this last treatment!"

Because of the sores, Dr. Guinan couldn't administer the Methotrexate, and as Dr. Guinan indicated, Mary Ellen had been very nearly on schedule. "This last treatment isn't that vital." And so we were done.

Our joy was indescribable, as we cried with Mary Ellen that it was over: all the vomiting, the blood tests, the IVs, the poking and prodding, the hospital beds, and all the side effects of this thirteen-month ordeal. I called Jimmy at the electric company and we rejoiced over the phone. Dr. Guinan told us to make an appointment for a month's time, and then we were off. On the return trip Holly, Mary Ellen, and I celebrated with a lunch at the Legal Sea Foods restaurant in Chestnut Hill, one of our very favorite places.

Now, with the protocol finished, Mary Ellen, reflecting upon these past thirteen months, indicated that there were two advantages to the chemo: "Losing excess weight so I can fit into size eight pants, and no more zits!" From the first treatment, Mary Ellen's face had suddenly cleared of all teenage acne, and she became proud of her beautiful complexion. Despite the side effects of the drugs, Mary Ellen always concerned herself with her appearance. Without hair, she still managed to look great. Even recovering from strenuous treatments, she appeared to be feeling fit. I'm certain that her upbeat attitude had a great deal to do with maintaining a bright smile rather than a bedraggled appearance. Teresa Gulotta, a close friend, captured Mary Ellen's devilish spirit regarding her bald head as she wrote, "Driving to Pittsfield, Mel would have no hair, so she'd moon people with her head, slipping down the bandanna, exposing her shiny bald head to those who chose to stare. Then she'd snicker as if in victory." Teresa continued, "She always seemed to have a comeback, no matter what. When she came to Tucson to visit, we were in my office when an agent [Teresa is a DEA with the FBI] asked Mel what she had done to her leg to cause the use of a cane. Mary Ellen smugly passed it off as roughhousing with me, which caused us all to laugh."

Usually when asked about her leg and why the crutches or cane, Mary Ellen would respond, "You *really* don't want to know." Occasionally people became insistent, and then Mary Ellen would tell the truth. She always felt bad under these circumstances because those who had insisted then felt terrible.

Now as we rejoiced that the chemo was over and done with, Mary Ellen brought up the subject of the party—the biggest party ever—to celebrate the end of chemo. As the guest list grew, we wondered where we could hold it. Katherine worked at the Weathervane Inn in South Egremont and the Murphys, the owners,

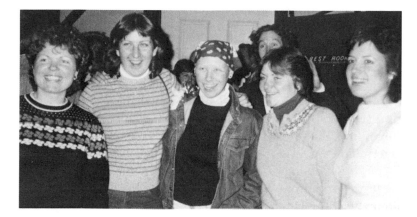

Kathi, Ellen Z, Mary Ellen, Mary Beth, Diane
—the nurses from Division 36

were good friends. On the inn grounds stood the Robbie Burns Pub, which the Murphys opened on Saturdays for dancing. They were closing the pub but agreed to let us have the party there. We invited all of the nurses from Boston, as well as the Rinkles, our relatives, Dr. Gallup and his wife, and many school friends, skiing buddies, and teachers: one hundred and fifteen guests in all. We planned on refreshments and a disc jockey, and Grandpa hired a magician.

The day of the party dawned cloudy, icy, and drizzly. Shelley Goverman and her husband, Barnett, had arrived the night before so they could ski with Mary Ellen the afternoon of the party. Actually, Mary Ellen taught Barnett some skiing fundamentals that afternoon, since it was only his second time on the slopes. After a few quick lessons, Shelley and Mary Ellen took off, leaving Barnett to ride the lift with whomever he might find since he did not have her expertise! Barnett found a very pleasant woman to go up with and enjoyed skiing at his own pace, not "zinging" down the slopes Mary Ellen-style.

Despite the weather, almost all of the invited guest came. Seven nurses from Division 36 piled into a van and drove the 136 miles to celebrate with us. The Rinkles came, as did my sister's family from New York. Dr. Gallup and his wife were unable to attend because of the weather but, a few days later, Mary Ellen received a handmade Valentine card from him, with the greeting: "Good-bye Chemo, Hello Hair." This thoughtful gesture is indicative of the kind of doctor we were fortunate to have as a pediatrician—a concerned, sensitive, caring person.

Jim Jr. and our good friend Brian Callahan, who gave us all corsages, took care of the bartending and the refreshments. Jimmy, who doesn't usually feel comfortable in the limelight, was determined to introduce all of those who had helped to make the chemo ordeal a bit more bearable; particularly those who had made the trip from Boston. After these initial introductions, Jimmy addressed his next remarks to Tammy Jervas, Mary Ellen's schoolmate and skiing pal for many years. Tammy had given Mary Ellen a hat at the time of the amputation: a hat that was Tammy's prized possession. With the hat went the stipulation: "This is yours until you make your first run. Then I want it back." The hat hung on the doorknob, a subtle reminder of the fun times they had had skiing and of a promise that those times would come again. Since Mary Ellen had made that first run a few short weeks before, Jimmy returned Tammy's hat.

The party was voted a huge success. Everyone who came rejoiced with us that Mary Ellen had completed the protocol and that now our lives perhaps would slow down. A permanent prosthesis would be designed so Mary Ellen could finally exchange the temporary one for a better-fitting, more streamlined model.

Part 3

1

❦

THE COMPLETION OF THE PROTOCOL DID NOT PUT AN END TO monthly visits, blood tests, X-rays, CT scans (X-ray technique for detecting masses in the body), and bone scans because all of these were necessary in the aggressive treatment of the cancer. Each month we returned to the Jimmy Fund Clinic, usually on Fridays, leaving home about 6:30 a.m. and arriving in Boston by 9:30. Jimmy, Mary Ellen, and I made these trips together. The routine at the Clinic remained the same during the previous thirteen months: a quick check of blood pressure, height, weight, and then a blood test. After these chores were completed, we'd go downstairs for an X-ray; then quickly back upstairs to wait for Dr. Guinan to review the X-ray and give us the results. During the months of chemo, Mary Ellen felt protected against any metastases. Dr. Guinan once said, "Mary Ellen is at her best during treatment, because she feels protected. The treatments give her a sense of security against possible recurrences of tumor." Now that the treatment was over, we were happy, yet apprehensive.

Each month as we sat and waited for the report, our nerves played strange tricks. If Dr. Guinan were unable to read the X-ray immediately and we had to wait, the minutes dragged by and our thoughts always were the same—there's something wrong. Jimmy would usually go outside and walk up and down Binney Street, checking on the progress of the ever-continuing construction around the Dana-Faber. Mary Ellen might flip through a magazine, not really reading the articles nor really seeing the pictures. Sometimes we chatted with Carol at the hematology desk. The longer we sat, the edgier Mary Ellen would become. I probably recited hundreds of Hail Marys, just waiting and praying for the news to be good. Marcia Delorey, the pediatric oncology clinical research nurse assigned to the osteogenic team, sometimes stopped by to chat. Jimmy hated to see her come because he associated her arrival with bad news. A few weeks after Mary Ellen

67

had died, when we met with Marcia and Dr. Guinan at lunch, we asked Marcia, "Why did you seem to appear consistently with our visits?"

She answered, "I really wanted to visit with you."

Jimmy, however, still was convinced that her presence, since it often accompanied bad news, was an ill-fated omen.

As we watched out of the corner of our eyes for Dr. Guinan to come up the winding stairs from X-ray, we tried to guess the results from her appearance. A big smile with an "okay" temporarily lifted a burden that would be shouldered again in a month's time. During February, March, April, and May with the prom, and June with graduation, we were elated. We actually enjoyed these monthly visits to Boston—visiting Quincy Market; Filene's; Copley Plaza with Neiman Marcus, where Mary Ellen usually inveigled her father into buying her a sweater or a pair of pants; the Chestnut Hill Mall; and, of course, lunch at our favorite restaurant, Legal Sea Foods. Mary Ellen had put on some weight, and she really started to resemble her old self. Her hair began growing back, and we hoped that soon she could shed the bandanna.

During one of our monthly visits after the end of chemo, the nurses planned a champagne party to celebrate. This party had become a tradition for all patients when they finished the protocol. These were the nurses Mary Ellen wrote about later on, while a student at Springfield College: "They took me to baseball games and out to dinner. They ordered pizza and Chinese for me. I don't know what I would have done without their support." As we celebrated the end of chemo with all our dear hospital friends, we rejoiced, hoping this would be the end of what had been a most difficult chapter in our lives.

2

THE PERMANENT PROSTHESIS HAD BEEN PUT ON HOLD BE-
cause of the swelling and fluctuation of body weight during the
chemo. About six weeks after the treatments ceased, we reported
to the brace shop and to Sal for the initial step, the casting for the
new limb. This process took a few hours, but the time passed
quickly as we chatted about the new leg. No more heavy sock, belt
or crutches, but rather a prosthesis slipped on by using a light-
weight ribbed cotton stocking. When the stump was well posi-
tioned into the socket, the cotton stocking could be removed
through a small opening which then was closed with a valve, used
mainly to control the suction. We eagerly read the material Shelley
gave us to become more familiar with this beautiful new limb,
which would have a knee controlled with a mechanism so it could
be easily bent or held straight. In two weeks' time we returned to
the brace shop for the first fitting. Sal, who was very meticulous,
demanded two fittings to ensure a perfect fit. Finally, one day in
April, Sal introduced us to the new limb. Excitement as well as
frustration reigned as he instructed Mary Ellen in the proper
donning and removing process. After a few unsuccessful at-
tempts, *success*! The leg was on and suction maintained. Mary
Ellen, still a bit nervous without the belt, asked Sal, "Could you
please attach a belt, just in case?"

Sal agreed. He did, however, state, "Don't depend on it. The
suction will work fine."

Sal proved correct and in two weeks Mary Ellen begged her
father, "Take off the belt, please." Oscar, the newly christened leg,
emerged.

The donning of Oscar wasn't always an easy task. Using baby
powder on her stump and then the ribbed stocking, Mary Ellen
often had to try several times before Oscar was secure. Many times
she became frustrated and angry with herself because Oscar,
often stubborn, did not cooperate on the first try. After a few

weeks and after several visits to the brace shop, however, Oscar became much easier to handle.

Mary Ellen now used the crutches only in the evening after Oscar was put to bed. During the day, to make walking a bit easier, she used the cane Jack Lloyd had given her. Oscar was indeed the Mercedes of prostheses, as Sal put it. Technically, Oscar was a fine-tuned appendage with quadrilateral suction socket, a sash foot, and a hydraulic mach knee.

During the thirteen-month protocol, while Mary Ellen worked with Shelley, Shelley tried to convince her to view "Celebrate," a film depicting amputee skiers using outriggers. Shelley stated, "Mary Ellen always seemed to find a reason for not viewing this film. Either she was too sick, just didn't want to, was tired, nauseous, or not in the mood." Shelley then added, "I don't think she really wanted to see the film." However, Shelley continued, "In January of 1984, when she got her own outriggers and when she had made her 'first run' as an amputee, she then agreed to view the film." Reflecting on this time in Mary Ellen's battle, I feel this was a turning point in her attitude, in her whole being. She now seemed all of a sudden to accept what had happened to her and began to put her life into gear.

With the protocol completed, Mary Ellen emerged bound and determined to carry on with her life and to make the best of a dreadful situation. She had hated Boston and the hospital. She was heard to remark, "I don't care if I ever see that place again." After she discovered skiing was truly possible and that she was just as good a skier with one leg as she had been with two, her outlook became much more positive. Boston didn't seem so terrible now that treatments were over. It was now that Mary Ellen began to entertain the thoughts of a career in physical therapy. Shelley, of course, was delighted and urged Mary Ellen on in pursuing this goal.

As Mary Ellen became accustomed to Oscar, Joan Widell, a member of the physical therapy department at the hospital, suggested that perhaps lofstrends, the two crutches in which she could rest her arms while walking, would help with Mary Ellen's mobility. She wanted no part of these contraptions, as she called them. Even though these crutches would have made walking easier, Shelley and I both agreed that Mary Ellen refused to resort to these because the regular crutches appeared more athletic. People with athletic injuries used the regular crutches; whereas those with a definite handicap used the others. Mary Ellen never considered herself handicapped. She hated the handicap plate for the car, but we felt that sometime it might come in handy. It was a rare instance that she used a handicap parking place.

After a few more visits to the brace shop, Mary Ellen became very adept at walking and Oscar seemed to be working out well. While a student at Springfield College, she wrote a paper entitled "Amputations" for her Introductory to Rehabilitation class. In this paper she summed up her situation:

> The treatment that the amputee goes through after the amputation is vital. Getting the stump ready for the abuse the prosthesis might put on it is important. For example, it is necessary to make sure that there are no sores on the stump, that the bone has healed properly, and that the muscle has been strengthened and ready to go. The next few steps may seem minor to some people, but for the amputee, they are important. Exercise and strengthening the rest of the body must be done. The body is now compensating for its loss and it must be ready to take on the extra strain. Hygiene is also very important. The cleaning of the stump and of the prosthesis are also necessities. For example, cleaning the stump at night might cut down on swelling when the prosthesis is being worn. Also, daily care of the prosthesis will keep it in better working order and possibly make it last longer.
>
> Being an amputee myself, many of the issues in the chapter of our textbook either bring back 'fond' memories, or I'm still experiencing them today in order to keep myself in shape. One of the major points made was the actual treatment and rehabilitation of my stump and the rest of my body. Luckily, I have had very few problems with my stump in regard to wearing my prosthesis. There have been minor sores here and there when I have started wearing a new prosthesis, but they were quickly taken care of. Often, either the nurses or physical therapists will slap the end of the stump to strengthen it or to get rid of any

funny sensations. Many of my friends find this particularly strange, but I can still feel my right foot and can distinguish which toe is which. This is referred to as "phantom pain," and different people experience different feelings. Some have it with them the rest of their lives, while others have it only for a period of time.

The actual rehabilitation of the body can be very rigorous. In the past four years, I have been through many long hours of physical therapy both in hospital and at home. While in the hospital for my operation, I was taken to the gym twice a day either to work on navigating the stairs on my new crutches or to practice hobbling between the parallel bars. When I was discharged from the hospital, I was sent home with all kinds of exercises to begin the long haul of strengthening my stump. When I finally received my first prosthesis, which was only temporary until I finished chemotherapy, I started the process of learning how to walk all over again. It didn't take long to get the hang of my "new" leg, but that wasn't the end of my PT sessions. It wasn't until last year and three legs later that my physical therapist decided I was finally walking as well as I ever would. The rest would have to be up to me. I would have to continue exercising my stump and the rest of my body so that I could continue to get stronger and to eventually get rid of my cane. All summer I worked out at a physical therapist's. I would go three days a week for an hour and a half, working on my stump and getting in shape for the upcoming skiing season.

I can remember when I got my first prosthesis. I didn't want any part of it because it just slowed me down. I could move faster on my crutches and only one leg. After a while, I got used to wearing it and today I feel as if it is a part of me. Sometimes, I actually forget I am wearing a prosthesis until it comes time to go to bed and I must take it off. One of my friends even named my second leg Oliver. It's because of friends like this that I have an optimistic attitude and bright outlook on life and don't become depressed about my situation.

3

THE SENIOR YEAR AT MOUNT EVERETT WOUND DOWN AS SOFT-
ball season began. Plans for the prom were a number one priority,
and thoughts about graduation and next year were uppermost in
the minds of Mary Ellen's classmates. Many of her friends were
going off to college, but we felt, as did Mary Ellen, that a year of
postgraduate work would help to strengthen her academics as
well as give her another year to relax and to enjoy school and
classes. Berkshire School, a co-ed college preparatory school with
an enrollment of 425 in Sheffield, accepted Mary Ellen as a postgraduate student, awarding her a very generous scholarship. Here
she would join the ranks of about thirty day students, driving to
campus in time for 8 a.m. classes and returning home at 5:30 p.m.
after sports. Her Berkshire routine would be different from the
four years at Mount Everett since she would now be attending a
private school with a very different life-style from Mount Everett.
Classes at Berkshire took place Monday through Saturday, with
sports teams in action on Wednesday and Saturday. While at
Berkshire, she took the courses necessary for admission to a physical therapy program, since she had tentatively decided on a
career in physical therapy.

With the arrival of spring came softball. Katherine and Mary
Ellen were elected co-captains by their teammates. Mary Ellen
had been a pitcher for the team before her amputation and hoped
to continue in that role. Coach Bob Krol, recalling her comeback,
notes: "Mary Ellen worked out with her sister, trying to regain her
previous form. But by this time, Katherine was an all-star-quality
pitcher and I used her in every contest. Mel was delegated to a
backup role. The sports headlines featured Mel, and she achieved
some local publicity as she waited for her chance on the mound. I
never told Mel this, but before each game I would go up to the
opposing coach and talk to them about Mel. I told them I would
put her into the game when I was obviously way ahead or way

73

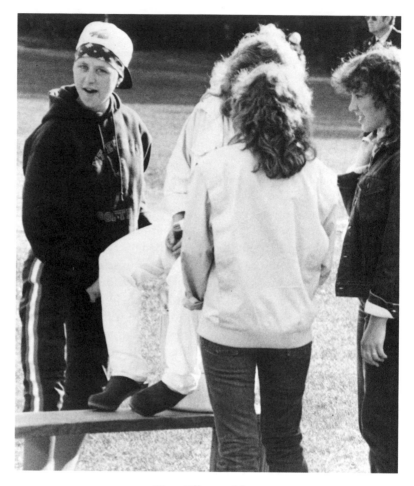

Mary Ellen and fans

behind, and if she did go in, please remember she was out there performing on an artificial leg. Halfway through the season, trailing in a league game by a good dozen runs, I put Mel in. The umpire stopped the game and told me he would not accept the responsibility if she got hurt." (The Umpires Association had contacted Jimmy and me and also our principal, Ray Chamberland, about her playing. We had all decided she would play and no way would we let them tell us otherwise. As Mary Ellen so aptly put it, "Who do they think they are? I'm playing and they can just try and stop me.") Bob continued, "I assured the umpire that I would take full responsibility, and the game continued. I expected only the best from the opposing coach—but was met almost immediately with a series of bunts. The game ended by our losing by over twenty runs. On the hour-long bus ride home, I sat in the stairwell where no one could see, and cried. When I think back to that day, I don't really know why I cried. Did I feel sorry for Mel—for the team—for myself? Was I upset over the embarrassing score and what the paper would say the next day? I don't know—but what I do realize is I never did inquire about Mel on the bus ride home. Had I done so, I would have seen that she wasn't crying; she was figuring how she and the team could cover those bunts. She had spunk! Mel did go back in other games that first year back as a pitcher, and each time she did, you could see her get stronger and more confident."

What Coach Krol did not know, however, was that Mary Ellen, the day after the disastrous game, confided in Kelly, crying, "I felt like such a jerk out there on that field. How could they have done that?" Evidently, Mary Ellen carried off her role and to the observer she seemed to handle the disaster. This is the way she wanted it. She wouldn't give the other team the satisfaction of knowing her innermost feelings, but kept her head high and kept on pitching until it was finally over. She did remark to us, "That was the longest darn game I've ever played."

Bob continues with his thoughts, saying:

I think that's when the team started learning the lesson of spunk! After she graduated, she'd return to watch many games, and as she approached the bench, I would get a squeeze in the back of the neck and a 'How's it going, Skippy?' I would hear her scream for the team over and over again. My last memory of Mel was sitting in the stands one cold, windy night at the softball complex in Pittsfield. She screamed and cheered the whole game, while others were complaining of the cold. About two weeks after that game, Mel died. This year, as in the year after Mel died, I keep feeling her presence behind me. I keep hearing her cheer for the Eagles. I keep hearing her give me the lesson on spunk—'Don't give up, Skippy; they can do it!'

Mary Ellen loved softball almost as much as skiing. For one of her games, several of the nurses from Division 36 made the trip from Boston. Even though she didn't get in the game on that day, we all enjoyed their visit. Grandpa and Uncle Frank Kinney came to a few games. They were very proud of Mary Ellen.

The softball awards banquet was held after the season. Bob Krol gave the awards, and again, when it was Mary Ellen's turn to receive her varsity letter, she was awarded another "Standing O." She certainly basked in the applause of her teammates and smiled as she accepted her award. In the spring of 1989, the Mary Ellen Welch Memorial Award was created. Coach Bob Krol indicates, "The award will not be handed out to the MVP—or even to someone who plays in every game. Instead, it will be awarded to the girl who gave it all she had, who worked to her highest potential, to the girl who reminds me of Mel—to the girl who keeps teaching me the lesson of spunk!"

4
❦

IN MAY, ED DAVIS, THE SENIOR ENGLISH CLASS TEACHER, PUB-lished a few outstanding short stories written by the class. Mary Ellen's happened to be one of the ones chosen, and I think it reflects her personality.

Me and My Big Mouth—by Mary Ellen Welch

A shot rang out, and then a figure ran out the door. I could not believe my eyes. It was Denise Sadera. She came running toward me, screaming, 'Mary Ellen, help me! The whole varsity baseball team is after me. They did not like the way I was keeping the book the other day, so they just started firing guns at me.' I told her to go and hide and I would take care of it.

Soon the boys, headed by Todd Ranolde, came running down the hallway. They were all yelling Denise's name. They came up

76

and asked me where she was. I told them I did not have the faintest idea. They looked at me in disbelief and walked away. Denise came out of hiding and asked me what we were going to do.

I said, 'Leave it to me. Tomorrow do not go to their game. There will be no one to get water, keep the book, collect balls, or tell the batting order. After the game, they will all come begging for you to come back.'

The next day Denise came back to me crying, 'Mary Ellen, it is almost the end of the day, and the boys still have not come begging for me.'

We looked down the hallway at the team approaching us. Their loudmouth spokesman, Todd Ranolde, shouted, 'Ha! Ha! Denise, we did not need you after all. The dugout was really organized yesterday. We brought out water, kept the book, and not one person batted out of order. We did not even miss your big mouth yelling.'

Denise looked at me and yelled, 'Mel, you jerk. Now look at what you have done.'

She started chasing me down the hallway, shooting at me.

The moral of the story is never help anyone with their problems because you most likely will end up with the problem.

5
❦

THE NEXT MAJOR EVENT BEFORE GRADUATION WAS THE PROM. This year, Wyantenuck Country Club was the scene for the festivities. Mary Ellen went with Duane Lanoue, a good friend and classmate. Her hair had grown back fairly well, and even though it was quite short, a wig was not in order. As usual at the prom, a king and queen are elected. Mary Ellen was voted first runner-up to the queen, Hannah Pedersen. After Mary Ellen's death, as Hannah and I reflected upon that moment at the prom, Hannah confided, "I felt so guilty that I received the honor and not Mary

Ellen. I felt I should not be there accepting the crown. I did so want the honor to go to Mary Ellen. I felt as if I were taking something away that would have been so much more special to her. Some others at the prom resented my receiving the award and expressed their displeasure, indicating they thought Mary Ellen should have been crowned queen."

I reassured Hannah, "Mary Ellen was just so delighted to share the honor with you. I'm certain she was suprised and happy to be second to you, and never gave it a thought that she was a runner-up."

How proud she was to receive the ovation from her classmates! What a fitting end to a high school career filled with so much happiness despite the burden of cancer. For these happy times, we were able to put aside our sadness and to enjoy the pleasant times—always looking ahead with a positive attitude.

The last event of her Mount Everett career was graduation, preceded by the writing of the class will. Since several of her friends loved taking apart her cane and using it for things other than its primary function, such as "hooking" people around the neck, Mary Ellen willed her cane to Mike Coon, who took great delight in "cane antics." Her bandannas, another trademark, Mary Ellen willed, for obvious reasons, to Edgar Davis, senior English teacher. The three acknowledgments she received from her classmates—friendliest, most cheerful, and nicest smile—certainly attested to her most obvious personality traits. Mary Ellen was a gregarious individual who seemed to know everyone. She was constantly waving to friends and acquaintances. This characteristic, which truly helped her and us to cope, often bothered Katherine when they were younger. Many a time she would tell Mary Ellen to keep still. "Don't be so loud" was her complaint to her sister. I thanked God often that Mary Ellen was blessed with this trait. Her ability to laugh and to mingle with people certainly was an advantage during her fight against cancer.

Kathi Kelly, one of the nurses on Division 36, indicated that Mary Ellen smiled even though she carried the "spit-up pan" upon arrival for a treatment. Kathy said, "Mary Ellen would vomit in the pan, and then smile her 'hello' as she arrived on the floor."

Mary Foley, the IV nurse at the Jimmy Fund Clinic, also spoke of Mary Ellen's smile when she said, "No matter how she felt when she arrived in the clinic, usually carrying her little white pan, she had a smile. After I put in the IV, which oftentimes proved difficult because of her veins, she'd say, 'Thanks, Mary' and smile." Even though she happened to be down in the dumps, she'd still manage a smile for those treating her.

After school ended in June, Katherine, Mary Ellen, and I planned another visit to Betty McKenna's cottage in Rye Beach. Jennifer Kinsley again went with us, and since Danielle was in the process of joining the Navy, Michelle Grotz took her place. We relaxed on the beach and had a great four or five days. Michelle, four years younger than Mary Ellen, had been a skiing buddy and school friend. Michelle remembers her friendship with Mary Ellen as a very special one:

When I surprisingly made the softball team, and when I finally made a base hit, I heard your voice, Mellie, above all the others as you yelled for me. You always cheered me on. When you came back from the hospital that day in December and sat on the bleachers at the game and yelled, 'Hey, Mitch!', followed by a big hug, I stopped worrying and feeling strange. Everything was going to be okay, you seemed to say, as you carried on. My most vivid memory of us, I suppose, is sitting in the life-guard's chair in Rye Beach. We were looking at the ocean, just talking. It was nearing evening; we were wearing sweatshirts, I think, because it was cool. Katherine and Jennifer must have gone for a walk down the beach. I felt so close to you—it was a wonderful time. Somehow we had gotten talking about your leg [prosthesis] and I remember mocking horror that this new one did not have a name.

The only reason the next memory stands out is because it is the only time I ever saw you really cry. Tammy, Troy, you, and I were all scrunched in Troy's little red car as we decided to go to the Alpine Slide during vacation after your graduation from Mount Everett. You hesitated, but only momentarily, as we all headed up the chair lift. We came down once and you had had enough. We all tried to convince you to go up again, and you protested, and somehow we pushed it too far. We should have just let it be. Previously Tammy had asked me if you had ever cried to me. Tammy hoped you felt you could break down and cry to someone, because all that time she had never seen you cry about the things that happened to you. As we spoke, I remembered all the times I cried and helped you out.

You were so matter-of-fact about the cancer. I remember going out to lunch with you, and your throat was a bit burned due to the radiation treatments you had just completed. I ate and you had a shake. Life went on as we talked about everything. Somehow you always had energy to tease me. But you'd always reach out and give me a hug, 'Oh, Mitch, I don't mean it.'

You are so much a part of so many of us and you are at the center of many of my memories. I speak of your laughter because I still hear it. Your laughter rang in my ears as I lit candles for you in churches and cathedrals in Europe that summer before you died, but your laughter is more vivid now. It is real and so distinctive because your laugh belonged only to you as you shared it with so many of us.

6
❦

WHEN WE RETURNED HOME FROM RYE BEACH, THE MONTHLY visit to Boston was in order. The last few reports had been great, but this time we were in for some unpleasant news, as the chest X-ray picked up a tiny tumor the size of a pinhead. Dr. Guinan and the surgeon Dr. Raphael Levey decided upon surgery, since the tumor could easily be removed.

As Dr. Guinan gave Jimmy, Mary Ellen, and me the news, we were all three filled with anger and frustration. After the long thirteen-month protocol, we obviously hadn't beaten those little cells, which had journeyed to the lungs. Jimmy vented his anger by kicking the trash can in the office. Mary Ellen was visibly upset by the news and also with her father's conduct. As Jimmy said later, "The amputation was behind us and so was the long chemo ordeal. Mary Ellen had been through enough. Why couldn't she begin to live a life free of worry and of concern? She had paid her dues."

Dr. Guinan gave us hope, however, as she explained the procedure. There would be no chemo at this time but rather a thoracotomy. Then she went on to tell us of another patient who had experienced many thoracotomies and had handled them all with ease. Here was the hope we needed. Knowing that others had beaten the odds gave us renewed strength, as we prayed that Mary Ellen, too, would win the fight.

As long as the surgeon could go in and extract these little tumors, there was hope. Even though we left Dr. Guinan's office facing an operation, we were not defeated. There was a feeling of optimism, since Dr. Levey had indicated the extraction of the tumors would be routine. The operation was scheduled for the first week in July. Mary Ellen's comment on this date: "I'm going to miss Grandpa's picnic." This yearly event was one we all looked forward to and one that we would sorely miss, but we knew there'd be other July Fourths.

Jimmy's actions when we received the bad news were understandable, since we had fought so long and so hard. Mary Ellen had suffered enough for any eighteen-year-old. He had watched over her during her treatments, urging her to eat, insisting that she drink plenty of liquids, reminding her of her exercises, and just caring deeply for her twenty-four hours a day. Jimmy's sometimes overprotective nature emerged in a paper Mary Ellen wrote while at Springfield College for an Introduction to Rehabilitation class in October 1986. The paper, entitled "The Role of the Family," included a personal aspect when Mary Ellen wrote:

At the age of sixteen, I was diagnosed as having Osteogenic Sarcoma, a type of bone cancer, and as a result I lost my right leg. Ever since that day, my parents have been behind me 100 percent. If they hadn't given me such support, God knows where I would be today. I also have a younger sister and an older brother who have been very supportive. While I was on chemotherapy for the first time, which lasted thirteen months, my brother took a semester off from college to help out at home or when I needed to be driven to the hospital in Boston for chemotherapy or to a nearby hospital for frequent blood tests. At the time, my sister was a sophomore in high school and helped me out tremendously. I may never have told her, but she gave me much support that really kept me going.

Once I was well again after my first (and as I thought last) bout with chemotherapy, my parents were right there encouraging me to get right back on my feet and be a "normal" person again. As the result of this encouragement, I started pitching again. I had been pitching since eighth grade and just didn't think it was possible to do it ever again. Boy, was I wrong! During my senior year, I was co-captain of the softball team with my sister and frequented the pitcher's mound many times. Another result of my parental encouragement was the year I started skiing again. I had been skiing since third grade and will admit I was a pretty good skier at that. I was very nervous about getting on skis, but my dad arranged for the proper equipment to be bought. Before I knew it, I was back on the slopes, skiing my heart out and loving every minute of it.

There have been many times, however, when I just felt so overprotected that I had no room to breathe. Coming to Springfield and getting away from home has been one of the best experiences in the past four years of my life. My mom has always been the one who tries to be the mediator between my dad and me. My dad, ever since my operation, has been worried about me twenty-four hours a day. He told me this once after I got a little annoyed about his asking me how I felt for the twentieth time that day. I love my dad very much, but I just wish he would let me live my life to its fullest and keep his worrying inside or get over it. The worst is going to the doctor's for monthly check-ups. Whenever the doctor tells me the cancer is back, he loses it; and once he kicked the wall and garbage can right in the doctor's office. I guess I shouldn't complain, but I do quite often to my friends, who tell me that I'm the luckiest person in the world to have such great parents, and then I feel guilty for my thoughts. I guess in time I will outgrow this feeling of overprotectiveness and learn to accept my father's ways of dealing with my disability.

In conclusion, I would just like to say again that if it hadn't been for the support of my parents, I don't think I would have the outlook on life that I do. I just hope my parents are always there for me whenever I need them, but that they will also understand that I need to lead my life to the fullest on my own.

The week of July Fourth found Mary Ellen in the hospital for five days while the thoracotomy was performed. Jimmy and I both stayed in Boston, taking advantage of Margaret Ball's hospitality. On July Fourth, Mary Ellen's appetite still hadn't returned, and she was feeling a little sorry for herself because we had to miss the picnic. The dietician stopped by to check on Mary Ellen's appetite and brought her a huge dish of fresh strawberries, Mary Ellen's favorite fruit. This thoughtful act perked up her spirits enormously. After the five days she was discharged, looking great and ready again to resume all activities, or almost all. Despite the IVs and chest tubes, Mary Ellen never ceased to amaze the hospital staff regarding her ability to bounce back so quickly. She usually managed to look healthy and bright upon discharge. She used to say, "I'm a good advertisement for this place. One look at me leaving and you'd think it was a health club!"

A month after the operation, we all enjoyed a family vacation at the Lighthouse Inn in West Dennis on the Cape. With the next school year bringing Jim Jr.'s graduation from SUNY, Katherine's from Mount Everett, and Mary Ellen's from Berkshire School, we had felt this might be the last time for a family vacation. We spent five great days enjoying the delicious food, the beach, and the sun, tennis and golf. We laughed a great deal and had a relaxing few days. When we returned home, it was time to return to school and to our jobs.

7
❧

SEPTEMBER SAW MARY ELLEN BEGIN HER POSTGRADUATE YEAR at Berkshire. We spent a few days clothes shopping, since the dress code at Berkshire did not include jeans and rugbys, but instead skirts, dress pants, blazers, dresses, and stockings. Mary Ellen was heard to comment early in the year at Berkshire, "When I finish here, it will be a long time before I wear a skirt again!"

I think she was becoming a bit nervous about Bershire. I know I was. The kids at Mount Everett had accepted Mary Ellen; the teachers all knew her and she never, never had a moment's unrest there. Now she would enter the world of the preppies. Our one wish was that the students and faculty would accept her for herself.

In September, before classes began, Mary Ellen wrote to her good friend Denise Sadera.

> *Dear Denise,*
>
> *Hi there, how goes everything? It sounds like from your letter that you are having a blast. How are your classes going? Mine haven't started yet. Orientation is Sunday and classes start Monday. My whole schedule has been changed. In order to get into a physical therapy school, you have to take physics. Then I find out if you haven't had trigonometry along with physics, you have to take that also. I guess I'm in for a hard year.*
>
> *Not much going on here. Everybody has left me. The hardest person to say goodbye to was Tammy Jervas. I wasn't even here to say goodbye to Laurie. I had to go to Boston and forgot that Laurie was leaving the same day. Now all I have left is Danielle, and she is leaving also. She is moving to Virginia. I'm going to miss her very much. Well, I hope everything continues to go well and keep your nose to the grindstone. Take care and write back when you have the time,*
>
> > *Love,*
> > *Mary Ellen*

Jeanette Cooper, the athletic director at Berkshire, indicated the excitement she felt upon discovering that Mary Ellen had enrolled at Berkshire. Jeanette said, "For those of us who knew Mary Ellen, we were so excited to have her here because we knew what she would do. Many faculty didn't know her, but there was an electric response from those of us who did know her. We told them, 'Wait until you meet this kid!' Once she was here, it was infectious, her presence. She touched so many lives here, many of whom she wasn't even aware. Her smile, her enthusiasm and zest for life—she just was not going to have any differences interfere. The first day she walked onto the hockey field, she took control based on what she knew she could do and would do. She used the cane and all, but she didn't go around saying what was wrong. It wasn't a secret, and if someone asked, as Wendy Jordan did, what was wrong, Mary Ellen would matter-of-factly tell the situation. Her frankness was what made this instant friendship between Wendy and Mary Ellen. There was always a seriousness about her, about getting the job done, about getting done whatever was expected of her. I'd love to be able to tell you she complained a lot and everything, but I can't. Did she ever have a bad day? Sure. She'd come up here to the office and sit, plop down and say this and that and the other . . . and go on and on."

Jimmy, Mary Ellen, and I reported to Berkshire for registration day. After the registration process, students had a picnic on the mountain. We returned home to anxiously await her call to come pick her up. As we left the campus, we watched Mary Ellen climb on the back of teacher Peter Kinne's motorcycle for a ride up the mountain. Mary Ellen, I'm sure, made the best of her arrival with this grand entrance.

Nancy Duryee, a Spanish teacher at the school who lived on the campus and whose children Mary Ellen had babysat for, became her advisor. Mary Ellen could go there after class just to rest and relax. Jeanette Cooper knew Mary Ellen had enjoyed playing field hockey when Mount Everett had a team, so she invited her to manage the team. The semester seemed to be going well, as Mary Ellen enjoyed classes and getting acquainted with the students.

8
❦

OUR LIVES WERE GOING ALONG QUITE SMOOTHLY WHEN WE went to Boston for the November checkup. For the second time, tumors were picked up in the lungs. We observed, "Novembers haven't been our months." Again her life would be interrupted by either chemo or an operation. We had truly prayed that there would be smooth sailing and that all operations and chemo treatments were behind us. Again we accepted the inevitable and prayed that all would go well with whatever plan of attack Dr. Guinan might suggest. However, the thoughts of having to undergo more chemo or another thoracotomy were unbearable.

Dr. Guinan, I'm certain, was prepared when and if there were a relapse. Now she discussed with Mary Ellen and us a new drug, Ifosfamide, which had met with some success in Europe, but which was still in the experimental stages in this country. Knowing that whatever Dr. Guinan suggested in the way of treatment had been discussed with others at the Dana-Farber before being presented to us, and knowing that Dr. Guinan was prepared to do whatever was medically possible to help Mary Ellen, we agreed to the Ifosfamide. After the administering of the Ifosfamide, the drug Mesna would be given to decrease the likelihood of bladder damage. The entire treatment would take five or six days. Again we felt fortunate that Dr. Guinan, and all of the others at the Dana-Farber who were consulted, were deeply committed to doing their utmost to help Mary Ellen.

Since she fit the criteria for Ifosfamide, treatment would begin as soon as possible. There would be hair loss again and nausea, but the advantages of the protocol—the possibility that it would attack the cancer cells and destroy them—far outweighed these disadvantages. After the sessions—there would be five of them—a thoracotomy would be in order to remove the tumors and to determine whether or not the drug had been successful.

As we prepared for hospitalization for the first treatment in November, we discovered that Jimmy's Blue Cross policy did not recognize treatment with experimental drugs. Therefore, Blue Cross informed us that they would not pay for Mary Ellen's admission to the hospital. Each session would cost about $3,000. At first we panicked and had no idea where to turn. We were certain, however, of one thing: Mary Ellen would have the treatment regardless. The hospital assured us they would never turn away a patient in need of treatment. The Dana-Farber indicated it would finance the first one until we could investigate other areas of payment. Jimmy's employer, the New England Electric Company, upon being apprised of our situation, indicated that it would pay for Mary Ellen's admission to the hospital. They indicated also that they would take care of all Ifosfamide treatments. This was such a great relief for us and is indicative of just one more good deed done for us by people who cared.

I arranged to take five days from my classroom duties to stay with Mary Ellen, since Dr. Guinan had said that perhaps the nausea would not be as severe with this drug as it had been with the former protocol. We planned that my part would be that of tutor, and we went off with a few school assignments. During the treatment Mary Ellen tried to concentrate on her studies, but to no avail. She was very sleepy and just a bit nauseous, so we didn't accomplish what we had set out to do. We decided that since all of the other treatments would probably go the same way, I needn't play the part of tutor.

While Mary Ellen was confined for the chemo, the field hockey team ended their season and planned a "team feed" at Jeanette's home. The team discussed postponing the "feed" until Mary Ellen could come. As Jeanette said, "There was no way they were going to have it without her. I mean, we're talking an hour at my house, Friday night pizza. It was her . . . having her around, having her a part. How much she gave to them."

After five days in the hospital, she returned home and back to school. She worked diligently to catch up on her assignments, and again the Berkshire teachers were as helpful as those at Mount Everett had been. They gave her the extra time she needed to complete the work she had missed. With the onset of chemo, she again experienced hair loss.

One day she arrived at school with her bandanna. After classes, she reported what one of the boys in her geometry class had said: "Who do you think you are, Aunt Jemina?" I'm sure Mary Ellen probably ignored his comment or came back with one of her own. I'm certain that when the young man found out the reason for the bandanna, he felt bad. After a few days of seeing her with her matching bandannas, the kids became accustomed to them and gave them little thought. Mark Bredenfoerder, Colin Cadogan, Anna Seidl, Wendy Jordan, and Sandy Smith were great friends, as were many other students.

The treatments occurred about once every three to four weeks. Between the November treatment and the one after Christmas, Mary Ellen worked part time at R.K. Puff and Stuff, Bob Krol's toy and hobby shop in Great Barrington. She had had fun working with the manager of the shop, Joe McDonald, who had been her jayvee softball coach at Mount Everett. After Christmas, Mary Ellen and I traveled to Boston for the second treatment. I stayed at Margaret's and spent the days with Mary Ellen at the hospital or visited a few friends in the area. As with the first treatment, she spent five days confined to bed or wheelchair and then came home.

School resumed after the New Year, and our routine was again pretty much established. Mary Ellen continued with her classes until the third treatment, the end of January. This one caused a problem that we had not faced as yet, dehydration. Mary Ellen had always worked hard at avoiding this by having a filled glass of iced tea at her side while reading, studying, or watching TV. However, she did dehydrate because of the excessive vomiting due to the chemo. Instead of having to return immediately to Boston, Dr. Guinan arranged with Dr. Gallup to have Mary Ellen admitted to Sharon Hospital, nearer home, where she would remain until the fluids were brought up to normal. After being admitted and while awaiting Dr. Gallup to put in the IV, she turned to me and tearfully asked, "Am I going to die?"

I had had no idea that she was thinking this and was stunned by her question. I'm sure she struggled with the fact that she had cancer and that she was aware of the odds for survival, but to ask this when it was the farthest thought from my mind shocked me. She had been through worse times with all the chemo treatments and had been sicker, but I am certain that as she continued to relapse, she gave serious thought as to whether or not she would have a future. I assured her that this was just a minor setback and that as soon as the IV started to flow, she would begin to feel better. Sure enough, in about three days she was back home and ready to get on with her life.

The Ifosfamide treatments ended in February, and then the

thoracotomy was in order to determine the status of the tumors. By the end of February everything was over and done with, and we heard the good news that the tumors were dead. This was great news because it indicated that the drug had done its job. All of a sudden the hair loss and all of the other side effects were minimized as we rejoiced that all was well again. Now we could only hope and pray that the chemo had taken care of any other cells that may have been working their way toward the lungs.

9
❧

AFTER THE IFOSFAMIDE TREATMENTS AND THE THORACOTOMY, Shelley, Joan Widell, and Sal LaBella decided that Mary Ellen should have a new socket for Oscar. Because of the weight fluctuation during the chemo and other bodily changes, Oscar needed some repair work. In order to get the best of fits, Sal decided to wait until June to cast. Sal had moved from Boston to Springfield, where he had opened his own office. This was indeed a blessing for us, since his office would only be an hour and a quarter from Sheffield. The new prosthesis would be ready for Mary Ellen when she began her college career at Springfield College in August and would be christened Oliver by her friends. Oscar became a substitute for as Sal so aptly said, "Everyone needs two legs."

In a paper entitled "Osteogenic Sarcoma" written for her Pediatric Rehabilitation class at Springfield College, Mary Ellen discussed the prosthesis.

One of the most important aspects of an amputee's rehabilitation process is the proper fitting and obtaining of a prosthesis. The actual fitting of the leg does not take place until chemotherapy has been finished and the stump has shrunk to its final size. . . . The most common and preferred A/K (above-the-knee) socket is the total contact quadrilateral socket. A depression in the anterior wall of the quadrilateral socket supports the soft tissue and holds the stump so that the patient's "ischial tuberosity" (back of pelvic bone) can "sit" on top of the posterior wall of the socket. There are many different kinds of knee joints. Some can be fit with a single axis that has a free swinging joint or others can be fit with a hydraulic knee that provides different levels of friction. (Stolov, p. 182)

Prosthetic checkups are usually done by the physical therapist, often with the prosthetist and other team members. During this time, the socket can be checked to make sure that there is total contact in the socket, adequacy of suspension, proper weight distribution to the prosthesis and careful attention to alignment. Cane support is usually needed for some assistance, but eventually no assistance should be needed. (Stolov. p. 184)*

Mary Ellen had the new prosthesis to look forward to, as Sal assured her that this one would be far superior to Oscar. In the meantime, there were three more months of school before her graduation from Berkshire.

With all that Mary Ellen had encountered since the diagnosis, she often said, "I have lots of material for essays and term papers." Many of her classes while at Springfield College zeroed in on the problems she had encountered. Jimmy and I twice lent our expertise to interviews by Mary Ellen's friends for their classes.

---

* Walter C. Stolov, *Handbook of Severe Disability: A Text for Rehabilitation Counselors, Other Vocational Practitioners, and Allied Health Professionals* (Library of Congress), pp. 182, 184.

10

🍂

AFTER THIS LAST OPERATION IN FEBRUARY, BERKSHIRE SCHOOL went on vacation for the month of March. With a month off from classes, Mary Ellen was able to catch up on her missing assignments so she'd be ready for classes in April. Since she hoped to play softball at Berkshire, she could work out and practice in the gym with the coach, Bill Gulotta. All in all, it was a month well spent and Mary Ellen was ready when school resumed. She still wore the bandannas, but her hair was growing back, and by June and graduation, we were sure she'd have her beautiful hair again.

That spring, Jimmy bought a second-hand Ford truck from Sheffield Police Chief Jim McGarry. Jim Jr., Mary Ellen, and Katherine nicknamed it the "Orange Pumpkin." Mary Ellen had bought a Berkshire School sticker for the car, but Jimmy put it on the truck. She was really dismayed as she exclaimed, "Why did you do that? I meant it for the car." How she hated to be picked up in the orange pumpkin, which Jimmy occasionally drove to the school when classes and sports were finished! Quickly she'd get in and slouch way down so none of her Berkshire friends would see her driving off in the pumpkin.

One afternoon as they were leaving campus, the truck ran out of gas. Luckily, the head groundskeeper came by with the loan of some gas. Mary Ellen was mortified to think she'd have to sit in the truck, stationary on the main drive, while her father hiked to town for gas. Another time, the shifting mechanism failed and Jimmy had to drive through campus in first gear, traveling all of five miles per hour. When they arrived home, Mary Ellen again exclaimed, "I've never been so mortified and embarrassed."

Many a morning Katherine and I waited for Mary Ellen to finish dressing so Katherine could drive her to Berkshire, me to Mount Everett, and then go on to Berkshire Community College for her classes. Mary Ellen's having to wear panty hose and skirts sometimes caused minor delays in our schedule, especially if she were all ready and then noticed a slight run in the panty hose. She'd stomp upstairs, quickly change hose, and then back downstairs and off to school. Sometimes tempers frayed a bit in the mornings as we got ready for our day. She must have gone through a hundred pairs of panty hose that year. After a while, if I noticed a run, I wouldn't say anything as we'd go off to school. Katherine, too, learned to play this game. Then when Mary Ellen arrived home later in the afternoon, she would say angrily, "Why didn't you tell me I had a run?"

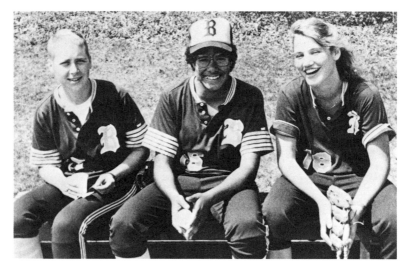

Mary Ellen, Ruthie, Jen—Berkshire School Softball

The last event before graduation was softball season. Berkshire experienced a good season under the coaching of Bill Gulotta and Chris Coenen. The girls on the team supported Mary Ellen in her pitching efforts as she had been supported by the Mount Everett team the previous year. When Mary Ellen told Coach Gulotta about her embarrassing performance during a particular game the preceding year, he and the team developed a strategy if this occurred. Everyone told her, "Don't worry. We have everything under control." They were a great bunch and we delighted in entertaining them, along with the coaches and their families, at a picnic after the season ended.

Bill Gulotta called us one day in late May to invite us to the Spring Sports Awards Assembly. When the softball awards were made, Bill, after giving almost all of the awards, said he had one more special award to make. He spoke about the team player who hadn't been able to travel to interesting places during the spring break because of catching up with assignments and who had come to the gym several times during the month to work out and practice with him. Immediately it dawned on us that this student was Mary Ellen. He called her to the stage and first awarded her the softball from the Hotchkiss game. Berkshire had beaten their arch rival and Mary Ellen had played a part in the victory. As he gave her this memento, he remarked, "I'd like to award this softball to Mary Ellen because of the dedication, sportsmanship and courage displayed by her." As Mary Ellen claimed her award, the student body and faculty greeted her with a "Standing O."

It was indeed fitting that in May 1989, Jimmy and I returned to the Spring Sports Award Assembly as Bill Gulotta awarded the Mary Ellen Welch Award to a student, Samantha Burns, and spoke these words, which appear on the bowl resting in the Berkshire School trophy case: "This bowl is given in memory of Mary Ellen Welch to the member of the softball team that best exemplifies the dedication, sportsmanship, and courage displayed by Mary Ellen." And again, four years later, another "Standing O" for us, Mary Ellen's family, as we helped to present this award.

We were busy with graduation festivities, since Jim Jr. had graduated from the State University of New York at Cobleskill in May. Katherine was in the midst of final exams as she prepared for her graduation from Mount Everett. And on June 3, Mary Ellen would receive her diploma from Berkshire School.

The third of June, a beautiful, sunny, warm day arrived, and we joined the other families and friends on the lawn in front of the library. The graduates, boys in green gowns and girls in white, assembled in the dining hall, preparing to walk down the hill toward the library. Mary Ellen's friends Tammy Jervas, Kurt Callahan, Laurie Briggs, Duane Lanoue, and Kelly Milan, joined us as we waited for the procession to begin.

As we watched the graduates proceed down the hill at a rather quick pace, Mary Ellen slipped. My heart jumped and all I could think was that she had hurt herself and wouldn't be able to get up. We sent Jim Jr. running up to walk along the side of the path just to make sure she wasn't hurt. She had quickly gotten to her feet, however, thanks to the assistance of a bystander, and continued at a slower pace with the rest of the graduates. Mary Ellen always said, "When I start out to do something, I do it big." She had picked herself up so quickly that very few were even aware of what had happened. Later on, concerning her brand new, never-been-worn shoes, she declared, "I'm taking these off now and never wearing them again!"

At the graduation ceremonies, the prizes and diplomas were awarded, and then the time came for the Headmaster's Prize. As Bob Brigham, the assistant headmaster, described the students to be honored, we listened and then all of us together exclaimed, "He's talking about Mary Ellen!" Bob told of the effect she had had on all of the Berkshire community and praised her courage and determination. "Mary Ellen," Bob continued, "served, perhaps unwittingly, as an inspiration to all of her classmates. She has strengthened us all by her presence at Berkshire." How surprised and excited we were as she and the other recipient, Shawn Ingram, went to the stage to claim their prize! Mary Ellen's winning marked the first time in the history of Berkshire School that a one-year student was so honored. Again she received her "Standing O." Upon graduation, Mary Ellen also received an award from the Sheffield Kiwanis, the Earl Sutphen Memorial Scholarship for $1,000.

After Mary Ellen's death, many of the Berkshire School people wrote, telling of her impact upon them. Jim Moore, the headmaster, and his wife, Billie, said:

We were devastated that such a courageous young woman should leave us so soon, and that her great fight for life had fallen short. We were exhilarated that her pain was over and that you, and all of us, now have a new saint to care for her family and friends.

She is certainly a saint. Many of us knew that as she lived among us. Her impact on people at Berkshire helped us put our petty problems

*aside. Few people ever can have a living saint live and work with us, but
Mary Ellen was one. I'm so pleased we could recognize her at Berkshire
when she was with us. It was a privilege to have her as a student; she
graced our school, and brought a whole new definition for living.*

*In the past thirty-seven years, Billie and I have come to know out-
standing students, great young people, superior talents. What distin-
guishes our career above all else is that in Mary Ellen we came to know
a real saint.*

*Please know our sympathy in your loss, but please let us also share in
the great joy that you now have in Mary Ellen's final victory with Christ.*

One of Mary Ellen's English teachers, Elisabeth Clifford wrote:

*Mary Ellen has made a mark on my life, as a warm and gentle person.
I taught her in an English elective and we enjoyed getting to know one
another. She was a dedicated student with a quick smile and good sense
of humor. My main memories are of her smile, when I suggested an idea
that struck her in class, and when she stopped by the field hockey field to
say 'Hi.' I will miss her and am very glad I had the chance to know her.*

Shawn Ingram, who shared the Headmaster's Prize with Mary
Ellen, wrote:

*In all my encounters with Mary Ellen at Berkshire, sports, dances,
theatrical events, I found her an exceptional woman, full of courage and
life. I will remember her always for precisely these qualities.*

Two other classmates remember Mary Ellen with these words:

*Mary Ellen was a friend and an inspiration to all of us who knew her.
She had a dedication to life that I'm sure you were aware of, and because
of this, she made us smile when we were around her.*
Steve Kazmarek

*Mary Ellen and I shared some good times at Berkshire together. (We
shared two of the yearbook pages.) I'll always remember Mary Ellen's
positive outlook and the smile I admired; she was one courageous gal!*
Betty Adotte

After the ceremony, Wendy Jordan, a classmate who was quite
an athlete—and who, I'm sure, deep down Mary Ellen perhaps
envied a bit because Wendy could do all of those athletic things
that Mary Ellen would have been doing had she not become a

95

victim of cancer—spoke with Mary Ellen and in her own inimitable way said, "Mary Ellen, you've got balls."

Mary Ellen had had the strength to carry on in spite of no hair, bandannas, operations, chemo, climbing up four flights of stairs to class and then back down the stairs, getting to class on time, rarely missing a class or a day except when treatments made it necessary to be in the hospital. Wendy remembered Mary Ellen when she wrote to me in May 1989:

> *I met Nancy Duryee as I visited Berkshire and she informed me of Mary Ellen's death. I was completely taken back. In fact, I felt a deep-rooted ache in me that would not let go. The feeling reinforced in me the idea of the importance of keeping in touch with the people you care about.*
>
> *I loved Mary Ellen! She was an incredibly strong person with loads of compassion. She was a good friend to me at Berkshire, incredibly insightful as well. If only I could articulate the vision. She was wonderful! What a disposition! There are parts of me that are strong because of Mary Ellen.*
>
> *I spoke with Jeanette Cooper and I cried when I heard you had tried to get in touch with me. I was touched to the core. I have not stopped thinking about Mary Ellen and the Welch family. She is so vivid in my memory right now.*

Mary Ellen would certainly reject the thought of her being a saint, as Jim and Billie Moore wrote. How she would have laughed and exclaimed, "Who me? Never!" I'm sure the Moores thought of her as a saint because she bore her burden gracefully and without a whimper. This disease was her lot in life. She had accepted it and had turned her misfortune into a positive outlook. Her vocation for the time being was that of a student as she followed her routine to the very best of her ability, not wishing to be singled out for an award when this was her job, her duty. As her friends and classmates indicated, her smile was her biggest asset, and with the smile came her determination and courage.

11

WHILE A STUDENT AT BERKSHIRE, MARY ELLEN APPLIED TO and was accepted at Russell Sage College in Troy, New York, and Springfield College in Springfield, Massachusetts. She had been considering physical therapy as a career, but the more she thought about this choice, the more she realized that academically she really was not prepared to take on a five-year program consisting of many difficult science courses. Finally, Mary Ellen decided to attend Springfield College, entering with an undeclared major.

As we discussed these two colleges, I told Mary Ellen, "My choice would be Russell Sage."

She showed her determination as she retorted, "Well, I've chosen Springfield. After all, I'm the one who's going." It so happened that her choice was a great one. For the three years she attended Springfield, she loved every minute of her life there. Through emergency room visits in the middle of the night, radiation, and chemo, the faculty, staff, and students were the greatest, the most supportive. We never worried about her while she was at Springfield because we knew she was well taken care of.

After graduation from Berkshire, Mary Ellen worked at the Sheffield Cheese and Package Store, doing a variety of jobs. In the morning she worked in the package store and at noon went to the little restaurant and helped in the kitchen preparing lunches. We kidded Mary Ellen because this was her first real nine-to-five job. We really didn't think she'd last the summer, but she did. She said at the close of summer, "I didn't really like the job, and after a day or two I wanted to quit. But I decided to stick it out primarily because of the two girls I worked with."

During the summer, Shelley thought that Mary Ellen really needed a more strenuous physical therapy program than she was following, since she wanted Mary Ellen to be in top form when she started at Springfield. Jay Kain, a physical therapist in Great Barrington, came highly recommended by Sue Young, one of our

Berkshire friends. We made the initial appointment, and with Shelley's referral from Boston, Mary Ellen started a program with Jay. This proved to be the beginning of a great relationship with Jay and later on with his assistant, Tammy Gebo. Jay had graduated from Springfield College and initiated a program for Mary Ellen with the physical therapy department at the college. Mary Ellen worked with Jay for the remainder of the summer and then continued during part of the first semester at Springfield to work with the PT people there.

The end of August we traveled to Fredericksburg, Virginia, to take Katherine to Mary Washington College where she would begin her freshman year. Jim Jr., after graduation from SUNY, took a position in the landscape department of Ward's Nursery in Great Barrington, Mary Ellen, after we returned from Virginia, began to get ready for Springfield College.

Part 4

1
❦

MARY ELLEN PLANNED TO ATTEND PRE-CAMP, AN ORIENTATION
session with about fifty freshmen that took place four days before
the actual orientation for all incoming freshmen. A week after
returning from Virginia, we packed the car again, and off we went
to Springfield. Jimmy and I were very nervous about leaving Mary
Ellen there as the pre-campers loaded sleeping bags and gear into
the cars for their four days at the camp area near the campus. We
didn't tell Mary Ellen that we were more concerned about leaving
her than we had been about leaving Katherine. I'm sure she
probably felt our apprehensions. We hoped everyone would help
her out if she needed assistance. We should never have worried,
because a young lady, a sophomore, Chris Brighton, nicknamed
Giggles, was in charge of Mary Ellen's group. Giggles, who remained Mary Ellen's good friend throughout her three years at
Springfield, wrote about her relationship with Mary Ellen, especially during pre-camp:

> We all loved Mary Ellen and I don't think any of our wonderful
> remembrances of her would surprise you. Your love for her and your
> strong support made Mary Ellen develop to her highest abilities.
> I have never met a person with so much insight and genuine love and
> sincerity for people—until I met Mary Ellen.
> I can vividly remember the first day I met her with you and Mr. Welch
> as you arrived at Springfield College for pre-camp. To be honest, I was
> so nervous about making a good impression and helping Mary Ellen
> feel good about going away to school that it all went so quick. Mary Ellen
> had written to me and had openly told me about herself, so I was not too
> surprised to meet a person so full of life and love for the first day. Most
> students, like myself, take at least a few days to let loose and have fun.
> But Mary Ellen was right in the middle of the fun. She had a special gift
> that made other students take pride and confidence in themselves.
> Maybe it was by her example. The first night of pre-camp we have our
> first trust walk. Usually the students are blindfolded and led by their
> leaders for a walk in the woods and eventually end in a big circle in the

"pueblo." I asked Mary Ellen if she wanted to be blindfolded or not—actually, all the students had their choice—it wasn't an exception. Mary Ellen chose not to, but she said she would close her eyes. At this time, Mary Ellen had a new prosthesis and wasn't too certain that she could avoid roots, rocks, and stumps. We led the group of students through the woods, all holding hands. I felt the initial fears of being in a new place, with new people and the unexpected. I was a little nervous, but with my hand in Mary Ellen's, I felt relieved. I don't know if I could explain it, but it was a sense of love. I was careful to point the flashlight down at the ground for Mary Ellen and to watch for roots, etc. that people might trip on. Initially Mary Ellen had her eyes open, but toward the end of the walk she kept her eyes closed. She had trust in me so quickly. This was very true. Mary Ellen was easy to trust and put trust in others.

Throughout pre-camp, I tried to watch over Mary Ellen. I guess I felt a little protective of her, but she didn't need it at all. Mary Ellen was such a loving person with a great personality that she made friends readily. Within the four days at pre-camp, Mary Ellen had opened up and explained to others about her condition—never for pity or sympathy, but for the understanding of others. I think we all respected her openness because it made us grow and realize how much we take for granted and what life was actually about—loving each other.

After pre-camp, I can remember seeing Mary Ellen on campus—always with a smile. There were times when I wished I could sit down and talk to Mary Ellen and ask her how things were. But between both of our busy schedules, these conversations were few. I wrote little notes and put them in her mailbox, just to let her know I cared. But Mary Ellen had a sense of pride: she never let me know how she was really doing.

I can remember seeing her one day on campus, not looking well but still wearing that great smile. At times I can still hear her voice saying, "Hi Giggles," only to find out the next day that she had gone to the hospital. She had a great amount of inner strength and a sincere love for life!

I realize that her closest friends have seen Mary Ellen when she spoke of fears and discouragement, but for the time that I knew Mary Ellen I never heard her say anything that wasn't tainted with optimism and hope.

Since I have graduated, I have been removed from the campus and, in a way, have not fully accepted Mary Ellen's death. When I have a bad day, I think of her strength and optimism.

...Mary Ellen was a true representation of the values that

Springfield College tries to exemplify—optimal abilities for mind, body, and spirit. Of course, these values start at home. Obviously, your home must be made of love and strength from the grace of God. When I think of Mary Ellen, I think of an angel sent from heaven. She has strengthened my love for life and faith in God. I am sure that the many lives that Mary Ellen has touched will state the same. It's almost unbelievable to think of how many people Mary Ellen touched—sincerely and lovingly—within her short lifetime. She must be an angel!

. . . Since Mary Ellen's death, I have been able to deal with some issues with friends who have been diagnosed with cancer. It has been a growing experience for me.

Again, how Mary Ellen would have laughed at Giggles' description of her—an angel indeed! She was an angel and a saint in the eyes of those who knew her and knew of her struggle, again because of her acceptance of the disease and because she was bound and determined to beat it or to put up an extraordinary struggle. Mary Ellen rarely let the disease get the upper hand in these early days of the battle. She seemed to take the disappointing news of relapse in her stride and, after the initial shock, she bounced back with her favorite comment to Dr. Guinan, "What's next in your bag of tricks?" Dr. Guinan, until the very end, was able to put our minds and hearts at ease as she and her colleagues did all humanly possible for Mary Ellen.

Part of the application for pre-camp included an essay written on the topic "We as Human Beings Cannot Be Responsible for Certain Things That may Happen in Our Lifetime." Mary Ellen's essay told of her battle with cancer as she wrote:

When I was sixteen, I was told that I had a certain type of bone cancer and would have to have my leg amputated. I was told on Monday and a week later I was operated on. I then had to make a big adjustment in my life. I feel I have made out quite well. As a person, I value life more because mine may not be as long and as healthy as the next person's. You have to take one day at a time and have as many laughs and good times as possible.

I know I have fully adjusted my sails and the sailing has been smooth. I know what I want out of life and I know what I have to do to get it.

Her thoughts in this brief essay embody her philosophy after the amputation. The last two years of her life, she did have to adjust her sails due to stormy seas. But adjust them she did as she sailed along, going for her goals, whether they were completing a semester or just getting through a difficult day.

During the pre-camp days Mary Ellen received her nickname, Mellon. The nickname emerged during a rhyming game the kids played and also because she wore a favorite Swatch watch with a watermelon design. To all at Springfield—faculty and students alike—she became Mellon.

2

AFTER PRE-CAMP, WE MET MARY ELLEN BACK ON CAMPUS WITH the rest of her stuff and started to move her into her room in Abbey Dorm. Melanie Hallier, Ann Kondig, and Mary Ellen were to share a room. That day we met Amy Kissel, a sophomore, who lived on the floor and was at school earlier than most upper-classmen since she played on the volleyball team. Amy, tall and thin, resembled Danielle Cote with her shoulder-length, light brown hair and friendly nature. When Amy's roommate decided to move to another dorm, Mary Ellen called with the news that she and Amy would be roommates.

The friendship which developed between Amy and Mary Ellen was a special one. Amy became a friend in the truest sense of the word. She looked out for Mary Ellen as they shared some great times. Amy's family—Carole and Sam, her parents, and Bella and Barney, her grandparents—became Mary Ellen's family, too. Amy was a dynamic member of the Springfield student body, and through her Mary Ellen made some lasting relationships. Amy was always there for Mary Ellen, in good times and in bad. And as they began the school year, doing all of the fun things and some not-so-fun things, Amy and Mary Ellen grew closer and their

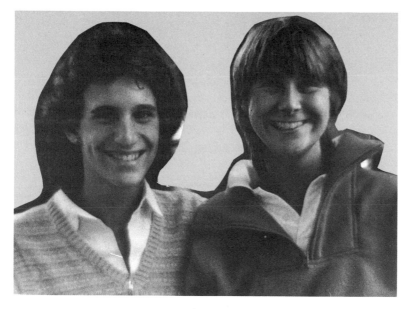

Amy and Mary Ellen

friendship blossomed. Through Amy, who was co-editor of the newspaper with "Jools" (Julie Gustafson), Mary Ellen took on the duties of circulation editor.

During the first few days at Springfield, Mary Ellen also met Wendy Cooper, who along with Amy became a very close friend. Wendy and her fiance, Andy, who we affectionately nicknamed Barbie and Ken, could be counted on for support, especially when the going became very rough. Wendy writes about her first meeting with Mary Ellen:

Upon arrival at Springfield College that day in August, 1985, I was a bit apprehensive, to say the least. But soon I saw a new sun rise. This sun had a name—it was Mary Ellen. I noticed a girl walking down the hall with not two legs but three. I didn't know what to think, let alone do or say. Well, fortunately, I didn't have a chance to make any kind of move. She said 'Hi!' so cheerfully and normally and somehow sincerely. I can picture her so clearly to this day. She was wearing a white "polo" (of course) shirt and white and black Bermuda shorts. Well, it wasn't long before she tossed her crutches aside and introduced me to Oliver.

105

Oliver was not your typical college kid (even for S.C.). Oliver was Mellon's $3,000 prosthesis. 'Why doesn't it have any toes?' was my first question. Mellon laughed and laughed. She told me later that it was my way of handling her situation that made me a special friend.

After I got Mellon to stop laughing, we were suddenly engaged in a serious conversation of how, what, when, where, and why. I sat wide-eyed and sorrowful as Mellon explained the 'Big C,' as she called it, and all that followed. I cried and so did she. I remember feeling incredibly sorry for this girl, and she was feeling sorry for me that I was feeling sorry for her (typical of the Mellon we all know and love!).

Then it was my turn. I told her the story of my life trauma—my dad's death. I'll never forget her words, 'Oh, if I could only change the way this world works.' Well, Mel, if only I could. Once again, we both cried, yet somehow my saga seems insignificant. It was then that I knew! My dad sent this 'sun' to me to brighten my college days and give me a precious gift of life—friendship. Well, Mellon, my dad sure knows how to pick them. Not only are you a treasure, but a true friend indeed. Mellon, you made my time at Springfield a time to remember. You taught me more than a book or lectures could. I only wish death had not been in the syllabus. Thanks, Mel, for teaching me how to smile, to laugh, to be happy and thankful for a chance at life.

During these early days at school, Mary Ellen developed a sore on her upper thigh which became infected, thus hindering the wearing of Oliver, her new prosthesis. Having to resort to crutches during orientation on campus was a difficulty but until the sore healed, she couldn't wear Oliver. Finally, a visit to Sal, who sent her to a dermatologist, resulted in a quick healing and again she had her two legs. This was the only time Mary Ellen ever experienced a sore on her stump. When I mentioned this to Sal and we talked about how well her prosthesis fit, he indicated that credit was due to the care and skill in casting and fitting her leg. We certainly agreed with him, because Sal is indeed a fine craftsman. He was always there for Mary Ellen, particularly as she lost weight during the treatments to come. Sal would patiently pad the socket to make a good fit while Mary Ellen endured weight loss.

3

❦

In October, the WBZ-TV network from Boston telephoned Mary Ellen about their annual telethon benefiting Children's Hospital. Libby, the head nurse on Division 36, had recommended Mary Ellen because she had dealt so well with her disease
by fighting it with us by her side. The telethon wanted to film
strong members of the Children's families to inspire and to give
courage to those in need. Through the patients telling of their
need for Children's and their reliance on the hospital's programs,
the telethon hoped to raise a record amount of money. We were
very excited about the prospect of appearing on TV. Mary Ellen
made all the arrangements, as it was decided to do the taping on
the day we were to go for the monthly checkup at the Jimmy Fund
Clinic. The brief segment would consist of an interview with us
and Mary Ellen, as well as a PT session with Shelley.

The day for our TV debut arrived. We went to the Jimmy Fund
Clinic for the usual routine. Since Dr. Guinan was busy, and we
were due to meet the camera crew at 11 a.m., Susan, the recep-
tionist at the Jimmy Fund Clinic, suggested we go do our TV bit
and then return for the results of the X-ray.

In the gym on the sixth floor we met Shelley. Mary Ellen
changed into her shorts, as she usually did for these PT sessions.
Only we forgot that the shorts were the black and white flowered
ones. These shorts made a wild combination with the aqua and
white wide-striped rugby. We hadn't thought about color coordinating when we met Mary Ellen at her dorm at 7:30 on the way
to Boston. No one really cared about the effect, least of all Mary
Ellen. The taping took about an hour and it was indeed a unique
experience. We felt like celebrities as the camera crew followed us
after the taping, making our way out of the hospital and up the
street to the Clinic.

With our TV debut over, we waited for Dr. Guinan to give us the
results of the X-ray, trying to forget that this was November and

Novembers had proven to be very unlucky months for us. We went into Dr. Guinan's office still excited about our TV performance, but knowing that Mary Ellen had experienced a nine-month remission, the longest period of time she had gone without a relapse. We were a little wary when we saw Marcia Delorey in the office because, from the beginning of the battle, Jimmy had associated Marcia's appearances with bad news. The news was awful. The X-ray had picked up a tumor or two, again the size of a pinhead, in the lungs, with one between the ribs, quite close to the spinal column. We sat stunned as Dr. Guinan reported the findings. We cried as she told us of the need to have them removed surgically by means of a thoracotomy. Not again. School had been going great for Mary Ellen. She loved her classes and the excitement of being on campus, making new friends and thoroughly enjoying the college experience. It just didn't seem fair. But again, with the original diagnosis came no assurances that there would be a silver lining to the cloud that hovered over her. We knew of the metastases and of their possibilities again and again. But deep down, we hoped and prayed that we had seen an end to these little tumors that kept appearing at very inopportune times. We know that God heard our prayers and that we did not pray in vain. He would give us the strength to deal with this as He had given us strength all along. Prayer and our faith seemed to keep us going, as we knew that the doctors would do all they could to help in the battle.

We left Dr. Guinan's office with instructions to return in a week's time for consultation with Dr. Levey. We had planned to celebrate our TV debut that evening by joining Shelley and Barnett for Chinese food. We did meet them at the restaurant, but our celebration was low-key; we did take heart, however, in the fact that Dr. Levey could operate, so all was not totally devastating.

4

MARY ELLEN RETURNED TO SCHOOL AFTER THE WEEKEND AND
spoke to her professors regarding the time she would need from
classes. Jimmy and I made arrangements with our employers to
take the necessary days. When we returned to Boston and met
with Dr. Levey, he determined that two thoracotomies were essen-
tial because of the location of the tumors. On November 15, Dr.
Levey removed two tiny tumors located quite close to the spinal
column. Two days later he performed another thoracotomy, removing a tumor from Mary Ellen's right lung.

Again Mary Ellen went to ICU with chest tubes from both
lungs. After a day in ICU, she was welcomed back on Division 36,
where she recovered quickly and waited for the chest tubes to be
removed. We had experienced the procedure for thoracotomies
since Mary Ellen had had two previous ones. The chest tubes
couldn't be removed until the X-rays showed no pneumothoraxes
(air bubbles in the lungs). At least twice each day as recovery
progressed, Michelle Briggs would come with her portable
machine to take the X-rays. We anxiously awaited the news as to
the progress of the pneumothorax. We had hoped Mary Ellen
could have been discharged before Thanksgiving, but our hopes
waned as the X-rays reported that the pneumothorax was still
evident. We were truly sorry to miss Dolores' gourmet Thanksgiving dinner, but at least Jim Jr. and Katherine went to New York to
be with the family. Jimmy and I stayed at Margaret's and celebrated Thanksgiving with a turkey dinner in the hospital cafeteria,
since the hospital personnel went all out with a turkey dinner and
all the trimmings. Finally, after a longer stay than usual, Mary
Ellen was discharged with a clean bill of health regarding the
lungs. She could do just about any reasonable activity and hoped
to return to campus in a few days.

As Dr. Levey checked with us before her discharge, Mary Ellen
kiddingly said to him, "Why don't you just put in a zipper so I'll be

ready in case I need another thoracotomy!" When she viewed her scars from this operation, she said, "I guess I'll never be able to wear a bikini."

Dr. Levey performed all but the very first thoracotomy and followed Mary Ellen's progress through the long struggle. After Mary Ellen's death, he thoughtfully wrote to us saying, "I am writing to you to express my sympathy on your loss of Mary Ellen this past June, and I want to tell you that she and you were an inspiration to all of us involved in her care. She was an outstanding young woman, and I know that only time will be able to ease your grief."

After the operations, Dr. Levey talked to us about the tumors' proximity to the spinal column. Because of the location, Dr. Levey could not remove as much of the lung as he had wanted to in order to ensure a good margin surrounding the tumors. Therefore, he and the other doctors felt that radiation would be in order to be certain that any little cells in and around the area might be taken care of.

We discussed radiation with the Brigham, but Dr. Guinan felt that if it could be done closer to home, it should be. As she said, "We want Mary Ellen to be able to continue with her life as normally as possible. School is important to her, so we don't want to disrupt that schedule." After some discussion, it was agreed that Hartford Hospital might be the solution. Upon investigation, the radiation team from the Brigham arranged an appointment with Dr. Joseph Cardinale at Hartford Hospital. Mary Ellen could begin during the Christmas vacation and continue after she returned to classes, since Hartford Hospital is just a forty-five-minute drive from Springfield College.

On December 30, Mary Ellen began the radiation treatment. Again our good friends came to our assistance. Beth Bartholomew and Ellen Emprimo frequently drove Mary Ellen to give us a break. She continued the treatments after returning to school, as Judy Meffen, the nurse on campus, arranged for volunteers to drive to Hartford: students, faculty, and secretaries took turns being her chauffeur. Springfield College people are caring and concerned for those in the college community. We certainly were

110

made aware of these characteristics when they all hastened to help out. Since the radiation caused no nausea, Mary Ellen was able to resume a full schedule for the second semester.

While in the hospital recovering from the thoracotomy, Mary Ellen received a letter from Frank Falcone, the president of Springfield College, illustrating this caring and concerned attitude that existed on campus. President Falcone wrote, "Please be assured that all of us at the College wish you well and are rooting for you. Hang in there and please let me know how you are doing, and take care." Mary Ellen's good friend, Jim Moore, headmaster of Berkshire School, also remembered her during this last operation and wrote:

Dear Mary Ellen,
I know of your recent operations. I also know of your stout heart, your courage. I only wish I had your stamina, your toughness. We all think of you, pray for you. You are such a terrific person; we love you very much. God often works in ways we do not understand, but in your pain and suffering, I know you accept it for us.

With support like this and the concern of her friends on campus and at home, Mary Ellen did indeed have a cheering section who sent their prayers to God, asking Him to keep her and us strong. She truly appreciated these thoughts, and I know she considered herself a very lucky young lady to have friends who deeply cared for her. She couldn't let all of these friends down, so she continued to keep up her courage and her strength even in the face of discouragement and bad times.

Early on into the second semester, the daily trips to Hartford Hospital for radiation ended. Mary Ellen again resumed her routine as a student and a vital member of the Springfield College community.

5

❦

CLASSES AND SOCIAL ACTIVITIES CONTINUED AS THE SEMESTER moved along with Mary Ellen enjoying campus life. The big decision at this point in the term was "Where should I go for spring break?" We were grateful that the Fort Lauderdale scene didn't appeal to either Katherine or Mary Ellen as they became involved in college life. Mary Ellen decided to spend the spring break in Arizona, visiting two old friends from Sheffield—Teresa and Lisa Gulotta. Teresa was now an FBI agent and Lisa a student at the University of Arizona.

During the third week in March, we drove Mary Ellen to Bradley Airport in Hartford for her flight to Tucson. As we saw her through the checkpoint at the gate, the buzzers sounded and everyone stared!

"Oh, darn," she yelled. "My prosthesis," she informed the startled airport personnel.

They scanned her with the portable detector and off she went. This incident became a family joke each time she flew, as we told her, "One will never know what you might hide in Oliver!"

She spent a great week with Teresa and Lisa, as they treated her royally with lots of sightseeing and fun. We were so glad that she had this chance to get away to a sunnier climate, to relax, and to renew old friendships before returning to school with the winding down of the semester, term papers, reports, and finally exams.

During the latter part of the semester, Judy Meffen, the head nurse at Springfield College infirmary, spoke to Mary Ellen about appearing as a guest speaker for the Springfield Chapter of the American Cancer Society. After some discussion with us and after some urging, Mary Ellen agreed. We pointed out to her that Judy had been a great help during her radiation period and that Mary Ellen certainly should seriously consider speaking to the chapter. The dinner was scheduled for June, after the completion of classes, at the Storrowton Tavern in West Springfield. Amy promised to come, and Mary Ellen also invited Tammy Jervas to attend with Jimmy, Katherine, and me. Channel 20 TV came to the house to film a short segment here at home, and they promised they would also film the evening of the dinner. Again we were to become TV stars. The speech was to highlight Mary Ellen's life since the diagnosis, her ups and downs, the treatments she endured, her existence and the changes in her life-style since 1982. It was during this speech that she said, "This whole situation has been a bummer. But it happened and I can't change anything. The only thing I can do is to look toward the future with a positive outlook."

The speech went really well, as I had assured her it would when she practiced it at home with me as the audience. After a few minutes she forgot her nervousness and was able to speak directly to her audience without reading from her notes. When we were introduced to the audience before she began, she stood up and insisted upon introducing Amy and Tammy, her two best friends, and made them stand up, much to their dismay. "If I have to stand up before the TV camera, I'm not going to let you two sit there," she insisted.

6
❦

THE SUMMER OF 1986 PROVED TO BE A MOST MEMORABLE ONE. After the speech and after I had finished school, we planned to go to the Lighthouse Inn, having rented one of their housekeeping cottages. Jimmy and Jim Jr. planned to come only for the weekend because of their jobs, while we three girls stayed the week. The weather cooperated, even though there was always a definite breeze and the temperatures a little cooler than we would have liked. We went to the beach and to the pool each day, improving our suntans and catching up on our reading. We had a really close relationship this week. It was also supposed to be our diet week, so we did almost all of our own cooking, rarely eating out. We did, however, succumb to the Sundae School, an ice cream parlor on Lower County Road. Despite our good intentions of shedding a few pounds, the homemade ice cream enticed us just about every evening or late afternoon, as we indulged in a gooey sundae or huge cone. We also played miniature golf at the Pirate's Cove, the most dramatic miniature golf course in the area. I realized that I was lucky to have had the week with Katherine and Mary Ellen and that they, too, were lucky to be able to share this time together. I know it comforts me as I look back on the fun times we shared or just the two of them shared as they occasionally went off on their own.

After we returned from the Cape, we were busy with the annual picnic at Grandpa's. Mary Ellen had gone to New York to visit Amy for a few days as soon as we returned home. They had a great time doing the usual tourist things in the city, as well as enjoying being with Amy's family at their home in Dix Hills, Long Island. Amy returned with Mary Ellen and stayed for the picnic.

At this point in the summer, Katherine had her job at the Weathervane Inn and Mary Ellen, as yet, had not seriously looked for a summer job. We kidded her that working at the package store the previous summer had been enough job for her for a while. One morning Susie Bradley, a neighbor, called to ask if Mary Ellen might be interested in taking care of Andrea, their special needs daughter, whom Mary Ellen had known and had babysat while in high school. Andrea would be spending a month at home, away from the residential school she attended, Camp Hill in Pennsylvania. Andrea's two sisters, Jill, the youngest, and Jennifer, the oldest, also enjoyed Mary Ellen's company. Jennifer, a high school student, often confided in Mary Ellen.

Mary Ellen and Andrea hit it off right from the start. Mary Ellen was very direct with Andrea, and as she usually did with her babysitting jobs, laid down a few rules that she expected Andrea to follow. They made cookies, especially the Rice Krispies marsh-mallow ones. Andrea loved to swim in their pool, so on pleasant afternoons Mary Ellen sat in the sun while Andrea swam. Mary Ellen never swam with Andrea. Perhaps it was because she thought that Andrea, seeing her minus a leg, might become upset. I'm sure she considered Andrea's feelings in regard to her swimming since she swam at Grandpa's and at the beach.

Jill and Annie (Andrea) liked to press the little button (as they called the valve) on Mary Ellen's leg. This little button released the air and was important to control suction, vital to the adhesion of the prosthesis. Annie asked a lot of questions, "Can I feel it? Can I press the button?" The prosthesis intrigued the girls.

One day as they sat by the pool, a mosquito landed on her leg, and Mary Ellen said to the girls, "Watch this. The mosquito died because he couldn't eat me." Annie laughed, thinking that was the funniest idea. The foot part of the prosthesis also intrigued Annie since it didn't really resemble a foot as Annie knew her own foot. Occasionally, when Annie asked her about swimming, Mary Ellen would reply, "Well, the next time I come I'll bring my things so I can take off my leg and go into the pool." Susan, Andrea's mother, remembers Mary Ellen's visits:

Mary Ellen entered our lives one day to help out and work with our special needs daughter, Annie. Rapidly she went from a sitter to a dear friend for Annie and a special confidant to Annie's sisters. Instead of going off to get some much needed space or a bit of respite, Jen and Jill stayed home to be with Mary Ellen, too! She touched all of us with her struggle to overcome this cancer that had a firm hold on her.

Mary Ellen's outlook on life was bright, her faith in God was strong, her desire to keep learning and striving for more was remarkable. When I find myself dwelling on the trivial or complaining, I try to remember to think of Mary Ellen and her family. You can truly feel fortunate if Mary Ellen's life came in contact with your own.

7

THE SUMMER OF '86 CONTINUED TO BE A VERY SPECIAL ONE
when Kelly and Joe Milan asked Mary Ellen to be godmother for
their expected baby. Corey Joseph Milan arrived on July 12, 1986,
and Mary Ellen was ecstatic. When I asked Kelly why she and Joe
had chosen Mary Ellen as Corey's godmother, she answered, "Joe
and I started thinking about godparents, and one day we both
looked at one another and without ever having voiced it aloud
before, we both said, 'Mary Ellen would be great.'" Kelly continued, "Mary Ellen and I talked at times and she indicated that
she thought she would never have kids of her own. We watched
her fight. When I told my sister, Nora, about choosing Mary Ellen,
she was delighted. I said that Mary Ellen could be around for a
year or for ten years. Who really knows? I just think that in that
time span she could do so much for Corey. She could have such an
impact and it would be so good for her. Mary Ellen is special and
we wanted someone special for our baby. Corey would know he
had a special godmother who had spent her life fighting."

Mary Ellen took her new role seriously and loved being with
Corey. She bought him his first pair of Reeboks, his first denim
jacket and rugby shirt. Corey's introduction to dipping chips was
compliments of Mary Ellen, as she showed him how to load a chip
with an excessive amount of gooey dip. To this day, Corey asks for
"chips and dip" when he comes to our house. Mary Ellen gave him
his first piece of bubble gum from the tub of gum she always had
on hand. Finally, she also taught him how to blow his nose using a
whole box of Kleenex and filling a wastepaper basket with slightly
used Kleenexes. When Kelly arrived to pick Corey up after he had
spent the day with Mary Ellen, seeing the overflowing wastepaper
can, she asked, "Mary Ellen, what happened?"

Mary Ellen answered matter-of-factly, "Oh, Corey's just blowing
his nose."

Every two minutes for the next few days Corey would say, "Blow

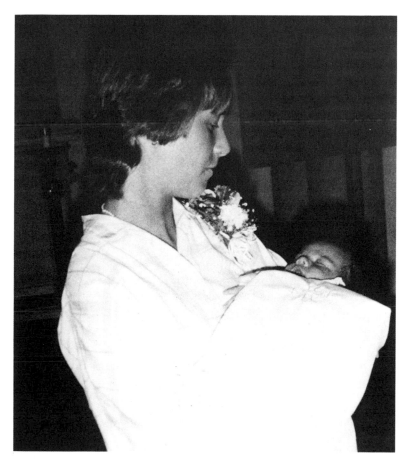

Mary Ellen and Corey

nose," using a whole new Kleenex each time. One day after Mary Ellen had died, out of the blue, Corey said, "Mel is my buddy."

During the summer, there were concerts at Saratoga with Artie Hebert, Troy and Tammy Jervas, Dan Andrus, and Betsy Aloisi. They always included Mary Ellen in their plans, whether it was a night of movie going, concerts, Friendly's, or just sitting around visiting: a great bunch of kids who were very attentive and who cared deeply for her. Besides the fun activities, Mary Ellen and Katherine enrolled at BCC, taking a course entitled "Human

Development." Mary Ellen needed the course for her major, which she had decided at the end of freshman year would be Pediatric Rehabilitation. She certainly was well qualified, since she had had much experience in the area of children and their needs. Katherine would not be returning to Mary Washington College in September, but rather would take a few courses at BCC and work full time at the front desk at the Red Lion Inn in Stockbridge. Katherine had experienced some difficult times coping with her course load at the college while she knew the struggle Mary Ellen was undergoing back home. Her GPA was lower than acceptable; therefore, Katherine had to take a year off before she would be received back in good standing on the MWC campus in September 1987.

One of the highlights of this summer occurred when Mary Ellen met Tammy Gebo, an assistant to Jay Kain, the physical therapist in Great Barrington. Shelley felt that Mary Ellen again needed some extensive PT work at home. Seeing Shelley once a month was not the ideal situation, and as Mary Ellen indicated, "Let's face it! I'm a bit lazy when it comes to exercises."

Jay gave Mary Ellen to Tammy for her own patient and merely said to Tammy, "Mary Ellen is an amputee." Tammy writes about their first meeting as she took Mary Ellen's medical history.

Mary Ellen started to give her history and continued for ten to fifteen minutes while I wrote. When she stopped, I sat a little taller, looked at her and then at my notes. I couldn't believe what I was hearing. She looked like a beautiful, healthy, twenty-year-old college student. I thought, 'How could this happen? This is not just an amputee. She has cancer.' As I asked Mary Ellen for her goals regarding the PT, she answered, 'I just want to get in shape. I need to exercise and to get rid of some of this flab.' As I listened to Mary Ellen, I realized I could help her reach her goals, but I wondered about the cancer.

We started with the strengthening, and as a new PT student, I wasn't quite sure how to do the strengthening on a leg so short. I attempted to put a Velcro-stripped weight around her stump. She let me try it a few times without much success, and then said, 'That isn't the way they did it at the hospital. They gave manual resistance with their hands.'

118

I remembered feeling very nervous, wondering if I were going to hurt her. Without making me feel any worse, she said, 'Just try to hold right here and you press down while I press up. I'll tell you if you're pressing too hard.' After Mary Ellen left that day, I had to sit down and gather my thoughts. I went home that night, and read everything I could find about her type of cancer, amputees, treatment, precautions and contraindications. Although I read everything, to this day I think that Mary Ellen taught me more in the first hour we met than what I learned in my entire first year of PT school.

While working with Tammy Gebo, Mary Ellen had gone water-skiing on Richmond Pond with Tammy Jervas, her brother Troy, and Artie Hebert. In reality, Mary Ellen was a boisterous observer from the boat as the other three skied. I'm certain she thought back to a time in 1982 when she was a mother's helper for the Duryee children on Twin Lakes in Canaan, Connecticut, and she had a chance to learn to water ski. She said, when telling us then of her refusal to learn the skill, "I didn't want to make a jerk out of myself, and I just knew I would since all those kids knew how to ski." We tried to talk her into trying but she was adamant. Now, four years later and with just one leg, the thought entered her mind, "Why can't I do that? If I can snow ski with one leg, I guess I can water ski."

When Mary Ellen reported to Tammy Gebo for her next PT session, she excitedly told her about the fun the others had had skiing. Tammy had friends who were great water skiers and who would be more than happy to help teach Mary Ellen. Tammy said, "If I get you into shape, we can shoot for the end of summer."

Mary Ellen countered with, "You really think I can do this, don't you!"

And Tammy, who doesn't believe in the word "can't," answered, "If you want to do this, and I really think you can, I'll find a way to at least let you try."

Tammy became a very close friend and confidant during this summer. Tammy herself was fighting a battle: to qualify for the World Triathlon Championships, the Hawaii Ironwoman. Mary Ellen and Tammy had set difficult goals for themselves, but know-

119

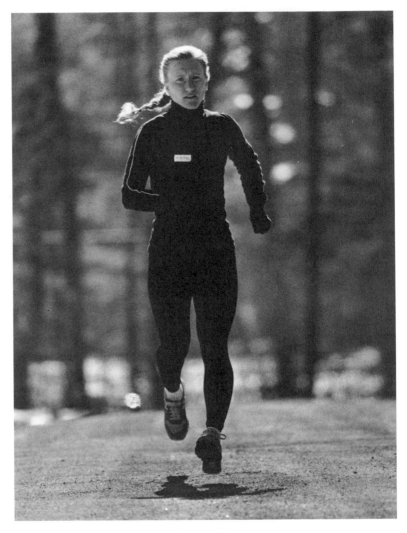

Tammy Gebo

ing their strong persistence and determination, they became each other's incentive. Tammy experienced one or two defeats on her road to accomplishing her goals, but as she unburdened her disappointment, Mary Ellen had these words of encouragement, "You worked hard and gave it your best shot. You'll just have to do better next time and try to qualify next year."

Tammy said that at this point, "If I ever qualify for the Iron-woman, it will be due to Mary Ellen's strong belief in what I'm doing. She believed that if you set a realistic goal, you should always go for it and never look back with regrets."

Near the end of the summer, Mary Ellen was ready to attempt the skiing. She had been swimming all summer in Grandpa's pool, had lost the weight she had wanted to lose, her flabby stump had turned into a mass of muscle, she had developed an incredible sense of balance by working on Tammy's BAPS Board (Bio-mechanical Ankle Platform System), and last but not least, her walking had improved 100 percent.

One afternoon Tammy and Mary Ellen went to Lake Buel in Great Barrington where the Raifstanger family, friends of Tammy's, were going to assist Mary Ellen's waterskiing debut. Jody Raifstanger explained the technique as they went into the water. Mary Ellen tried two or three times to pull herself up out of the water. She wasn't having any success when Jody slid into the water to assist by pushing up Mary Ellen's fanny. After ten tries, Mary Ellen broke the water's surface and was up on one ski, a huge smile on her face, maintaining her balance for ten seconds before falling into the water. She tried again three or four times, not perfection, but with a most marvelous sense of pride as she almost conquered the art of waterskiing on this first visit to the lake.

8
❦

MARY ELLEN HAD ONE MORE APPOINTMENT WITH TAMMY BE-fore our monthly visit to the Jimmy Fund Clinic at the end of August and before starting her sophomore year at Springfield. During this last appointment, Mary Ellen confided in Tammy that she thought there were some metastases because the scars from earlier thoracotomies hurt, especially in one spot. When we heard the news, therefore, that there were more metastases in her lungs, I don't think Mary Ellen was surprised. We were crushed. It had been a ten-month remission, and again we were faced with the awful news that she had relapsed. Would it ever end? Would it ever go away? It didn't seem so. We continued our prayers, certain that God heard us but not sure how we could deal with this terrible disappointment. But once more He sent us the strength to cope with the situation as Mary Ellen faced another thoracotomy. Dr. Levey indicated that he could remove the tumor, but he would also have to remove part of the chest wall, some muscle, and part of the lower lung and skin to try to make certain that no possible cancer cells remained. Again we were to experience the routine of operating room, ICU, chest tubes, and the last step before recovery, the X-ray to ascertain the absence of any pneumothorax.

Instead of returning to campus after a most marvelous summer, Mary Ellen, Jimmy, and I went to Boston at the end of August for the sixth thoracotomy. Again she took it in her stride, not whining or complaining about this recent twist of fate, but rather facing the operation optimistically, knowing that ten days after the surgery she'd be back at school, entering again into campus life.

The operating room staff knew Mary Ellen quite well, since she was such a frequent visitor to the third floor, but the person who knew her the best was Danny Tucker, the operating room escort who always seemed to be there when the telephone message came to escort her to the third floor. Danny, also a reggae artist who entertained us many times with stories about his record-cutting endeavors in Jamaica, arrived to escort us. The elevator wasn't working properly so Danny took out his key, saying, "I'll take care of this."

"I'm not really happy with elevators," I commented as the elevator arrived and Jimmy and I, with Danny controlling Mary Ellen's bed, got in. With his key, Danny determined we'd be next arriving on the third floor. Instead, Danny sent the elevator up and down, as the doors opened onto blank concrete walls, until we surprisingly arrived in the basement.

Again with his trusty key, Danny sent the elevator upwards,

laughing and telling us, "Not to worry."

Mary Ellen laughed as she exclaimed, "Maybe they'll put off the operation if we don't show up!"

Finally we arrived at our primary destination, the third floor. The nurses wondered why we were late, and then laughed as we told them of our misadventure.

Danny remembered Mary Ellen at a memorial service held at the hospital about a month after her death when he said, "I've come to know Mary Ellen many times. She was quite different. She had spirit. I've brought a lot of people to the operating room before but never one like Mary Ellen. She was different. She was happy. She was energetic. You name it. She was a great person. I wish the best that you, her parents, can carry on her dreams and her love." We all so much enjoyed talking and joking with Danny. He was a bright light on Mary Ellen's way to the operating room on that dreaded third floor.

9
❧

AFTER THE OPERATION, MARY ELLEN RETURNED TO SPRING-field. She had quite a scar on her lower back, and it was obvious where Dr. Levey had extracted the tumor, since that area of her lower back was now rather concave. Again she made the comment, "I guess I'll never wear a bikini. I'll have to be content wearing my old Speedos!" She felt great, however, and plunged into the college routine. Wendy Cooper and Amy had gathered her materials from her professors. Cathy Condron, one of the deans, had contacted her professors so that they knew the reason for her late arrival. In a week or two, however, she was totally immersed in the swing of classes and social activities.

Many of Mary Ellen's classmates and friends at Springfield College were aware of the surgery as they continued to support her during her struggle with cancer. She had a profound effect upon these classmates, and with her dominant spirit, she became a symbol of strength and courage for many of the students who knew and admired her. Karen Wooten wrote about Mary Ellen's battles:

I have known Mary Ellen since Day 1 of our freshman year. She was an inspiration to everyone she touched. She never showed the down side of things, even when things were at their worst. A feat such as that takes a great deal of courage, strength, and determination. Mary Ellen had the true spirit of Springfield College. The pride Mary Ellen had in herself has been a lesson to us all.

The characteristics for which she was best known, her courage, strength and determination, and her love of life are remembered by Malcolm Lester as he wrote:

Mary Ellen never ceased in cheering me up when I was down, or drawing a laugh from me when a laugh seemed impossible. She was special, and there will be a void at school next year without her. I will miss her and will always think of her fondly as I'm sure everyone who knew her will. She was a diamond in the rough and one who always shined even in difficult times.

Tina Margaris echoed Malcolm's thoughts:

There are a thousand things that I loved about Mary Ellen, but her ability to make other people happy stands out foremost in my mind. The courage and the strength that she carried throughout her illness was not only a deep inspiration to me but an inspiration to anyone who was lucky enough to meet her.

I'm sure it would make you happy to know that there is a little bit of Mary Ellen living in all her friends' hearts at Springfield College. I will miss her dearly.

Mary Ellen's presence on campus was like that of a major big-time celebrity. She took pains to know everyone and delighted in recognizing her friends and acquaintances with a smile and a wave. Alicia Medeiros remembers this:

As I think back to before I met Mary Ellen, I can remember how she walked around campus knowing every passing person and greeting them with a big, cheery glow and hello. I found her interesting because her disability was exactly the same as what my aunt had. That often helped me to understand Mary Ellen a little bit better. I often told her I was always there for her, whenever she needed anything. It's funny, she never did. I think that's why I admired her so much. She's with me every day in spirit and often I ask the picture of her on my wall what she'd do about a specific problem. I can just see her telling me what to do.

Mary Ellen had a way with people and seemed to encourage those with problems to confide in her. She took their problems seriously and genuinely tried to advise her friends which course to follow. I often think what a great job she would have done with young people in advising them and in listening to their problems. She was a true friend who would never divulge a secret or a thought given in confidence. It's no wonder she had so many friends, since they knew they could trust her and that when she knew strict confidence was expected, she lived up to this agreement. Mary Ellen enjoyed talking with the younger students, whom she referred to as "'Shmen." Sheila Dymes, an especially close friend and one of the "'Shmen," wrote:

Mary Ellen was a very special person to me. Even though I only knew her for a year, my freshman year at Springfield College, I felt like I had known her forever, because that's the way she was. She was a very comfortable person to be with. She was down-to-earth and real. As a matter of fact, she couldn't stand it when people acted fake. Mellon was also a very sensitive person. If anything was wrong with me, she was always out there, either to cheer me up or just to listen. Even if the problem was so trival, it didn't matter because she knew it bothered me. I was very lucky to have known Mellon; we had some real fun times together.

Mary Ellen, as Sheila writes, was not fake and had no patience with those who were. I do believe that's why she was so uncomfortable wearing the wig during hair loss. A wig was fake, something she was not. She called a spade a spade and really didn't care for those who were not up front and straightforward.

Julie ("Jools") Gustafson, the co-editor of the college newspaper with Amy—tells of a revelation Mary Ellen made one evening during Mary Ellen's sophomore year as "Jools," Amy, and Mary Ellen enjoyed a pizza. "We were just chatting, and Amy got up to go to the bathroom. Mary Ellen said she had something to tell me."

"I hated you," Mary Ellen confessed.

"Julie asked, "Well, why?"

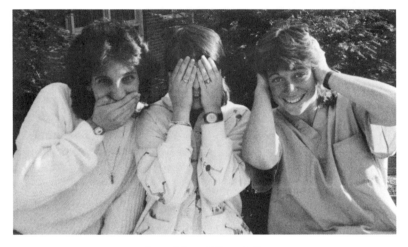

Amy, Mary Ellen, Julie

Mary Ellen explained, "Well, I was jealous because you and Amy were such good friends. I'm happy now that we three get along and that we're such good friends."

Julie continued, "I'm glad she told me that. It was the honest thing to do. I felt proud we could turn it around. Mary Ellen knew who she liked and she knew who she didn't like. There was no in between."

Again and again, the ability to look on the bright side seemed to be the quality that many of her friends admired in her. She was not gloom and doom, but rather sunshine and smiles. Peter LaMachia recalls this side of Mary Ellen's personality:

The most extraordinary aspect of Mellon's personality was her ability to always see the silver lining in every cloud—whether they were grey or billowy white.

I remember the first evening that I had been with her. We had been out with two other people and I remember how these people were complaining over frivolous things, but Mellon was just laughing and having a great time. It was not until later I realized that Mellon had cancer and had lost one of her legs to the disease. Suddenly, Mellon went from extraordinary person to patron saint in my eyes.

It was inconceivable to me how she could have such an incredible perspective on life, while at the same time she was losing grip on her own. No matter what the situation, Mellon was always smiling. I believe everyone has a purpose for being here. Mellon's purpose was to brighten people's days. And although her work was cut short, the outreaches of her work will be everlasting.

Mary Ellen loved a good time just like everyone else. She loved the atmosphere at Springfield and readily took an active part in partying with her friends as well as keeping up her grades. She was not a 3.0 student, but she did manage a healthy 2.8 GPA during her first two and a half years. She had a great sense of humor and wasn't adverse to playing jokes. Carolyn Grant remembers:

Mellon had a special something to her. It's hard to explain what, but anyone who knew her knows what I'm talking about. This special sparkle was seen in her eyes, smile, and overall friendly appearance. She was the type of person whom you are just drawn to without realizing it. There were the times we spent scoping men in the cafeteria and throwing food to get their attention. And remember, Mellon was a good softball player! The window-watching we did from my dorm window. Mellon doing a speech on softball, breaking the hall light and blaming it on me—"Carolyn, you did it!" Then there was the time stumbling home from a late-night party, or going to sleep on Lorna's couch, or the late-night talks about the men we loved who didn't love us. The list goes on and on. Even in the hard times, Mellon almost always stayed chipper. We never knew what to expect when we visited her in the hospital. It ranged from racing through the halls in a wheelchair, stealing doctors' uniforms, a tour of the hospital to find the gorgeous doctors, or feeding her Captain Crunch after a late-night party.

Through thick and thin, Mellon always hung on with hope and much more concern for her family and friends than for herself. It might sound corny, but through Mellon I've seen the beauty in life and I will never

127

take it for granted. I will never forget Mellon and the times we shared, for her love for us and her life will remain in all of our hearts forever.

Another close friend and dorm neighbor Janet Varell wrote:

While here at Springfield College, Mary Ellen was always there when I needed her. From day one, out at East Campus living in the woods for three days, to the last time I saw her, Mary Ellen cared for her friends more than herself. Mary Ellen was a social butterfly, no one can deny that, and she always wanted to hear how you were and never focused on herself, even when she was in pain. There were times here at Springfield when Mellon would come into my room and just talk to me and make me forget my problems. Whenever I saw Mellon on campus or on the floor of Abbey, I knew she would be there for me at the drop of a hat, and she still is now. Whenever things get too much, I think of the two sets of footprints in the sand and know that Mellon is still with me and always will be.

Janet's words illustrate Mary Ellen's ability to make others forget their troubles by their confiding in her. She rarely seemed to consider herself but enjoyed being a confidant to others. Another of Mary Ellen's classmates at Springfield, Patti DiGiovanni, echoes many of Janet's thoughts:

All my times with Mary Ellen were great times. She was one of the first persons I met when I came to Springfield. I never thought of her any different from anyone else because she never wanted it that way.

Mary Ellen and I spent two special years as floormates in Abbey, going to Friendly's and visiting her favorite guys, 'Good Ole C-1.' The guys of C-1 were always a great excuse for us not to study. My most memorable moments with Mellon were the times she spent just talking and spreading the latest gossip. She was always the one I ran to for advice and a little encouragement. I probably wouldn't have survived my freshman year without her. Somehow she was always there to cheer me up and point me in the right direction. It always amazed me how a person with so many problems of her own spent so much time caring about everyone else's. I still remember and try to follow her advice: 'Follow your heart. I know you can do it.' and 'Do what you think is best.'

Because Mary Ellen suspected that her life would probably be cut short, she, I'm certain, valued living more than others at the college. Knowing this about herself no doubt gave her unusual insight for a college student. Her disability, which she never considered a disability, she readily shared with her friends. Many a term paper or essay was written with her as the subject. She kidded her friends as they received their A's on papers devoted to her. "Where would you guys be without me?" she'd question.

When Mary Ellen first arrived on the Springfield campus, there were a few students with physical handicaps, but none with one like hers. At first, I'm certain that many students were a bit nervous upon first meeting her. Ann Hibbard and Shannon O'Neill tell about their thoughts when they first met Mary Ellen:

Meeting Mellon was our first encounter with a disabled student. We were unsure how to treat her and felt apprehensive at first. Through Mary Ellen, we learned to accept people for what's inside rather than their physical appearance. Mellon always brought out the best in all of us. Most of all, we think of Mellon as a friend, as she taught us the value of life and good friends with whom to share it.

Mary Ellen realized the value of friendship, as she appreciated her wealth of friends and considered herself blessed to have so many who genuinely cared for her. She, however, as all of her friends have indicated, could be counted on to be there when needed.

Kristin Mangiulli, who lived in Abbey dorm, remembers Mary Ellen in a special way:

During the time I was student teaching in an elementary school, the first person to call me Miss Mangiulli was not one of my students—but Mary Ellen. She screamed down the hall whenever she saw me, 'Mrs. Julie, Mrs. Julie.' The nickname spread to all on the floor. They say you never forget your first experience teaching—well, I know my first memories will be with me my entire life. Mary Ellen's spirit is with me forever and still remains alive with every student who calls my name.

Is it any wonder that Mary Ellen loved to be on campus? With friends who loved her and professors and administrators who cared, she felt at home. These relationships were a great source of joy to her. I believe the happiest years of her short life were those spent at Springfield even though they were also the most trying.

129

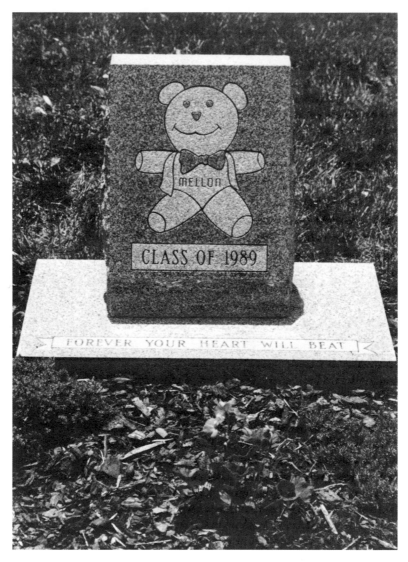

Teddy bear in garden at Springfield College

In May 1989 at the dedication of the garden and teddy bear marker donated by her classmates and bearing Wendy's thought "Forever your heart will beat," Dr. Robert Palmer, assistant to the president, spoke, "Mary Ellen was meant for Springfield. We have a special feeling; a special atmosphere. Springfield benefits from students with attitudes like Mary Ellen's. She gave to us perhaps more than we gave to her."

10
❦

DURING THE FALL OF MARY ELLEN'S SOPHOMORE YEAR, KELLY Milan and her son, Corey, spent a day with Mary Ellen at the college. She was so proud of her godson and couldn't wait to show him off to all of her dormmates. Kelly comments, "Mary Ellen sat with Corey in her room, and then took him down the hall to show him off."

The other girls wanted to hold him, but she refused, saying, "No. Today's my day. You'll have to wait until another day." Corey's visit was such a thrill for her.

The first semester continued along on a happy note. Mary Ellen did well in her studies and the monthly checkups went well, even the one in the dreaded month of November. Sal LaBella had completed her new prosthesis. His move saved us many miles of travel, since Sal was now only five minutes from campus.

During this semester, Mary Ellen's school friend from Mount Everett days, Todd Ranolde, called to tell her he had just been diagnosed as having cancer; a tumor was found in his sternum. Todd remembered this conversation: "When I told her, we cried."

Then Mary Ellen said, "You can't be a wimp."

Todd answered her comment, "I know, but it's not fair."

"There's nothing really fair in this world. I mean, you're one of the unfortunate ones," Mary Ellen frankly stated.

Todd said that Mary Ellen talked with him, telling him about the chemo treatments. She jokingly told him that she didn't think he could handle the hair loss. Todd, a good-looking boy, was always concerned about his appearance. In talking about his experience and Mary Ellen's part in his fight with cancer he said, "She helped me a lot. She was unbelievable. She was so strong, it was scary. She wasn't a wimp; she was very tough."

Mary Ellen's advice was to the point: "Don't get down. Stay in high spirits. Tell it you're going to kill it and that's it. Don't lie around. Even if you don't feel good, do something."

Todd said he used to lie on the couch between treatments; he didn't work and wasn't going to school. One evening Mary Ellen called him from Springfield and after questioning him about his inactivity, yelled at him: "Get up off your ass and do something!"

Todd continued, "Mary Ellen had a way with people. I don't think she had any enemies. I mean, even before she got sick. In school she was always a friend. She was someone you could talk to and not worry about her telling all. She was just . . . Mary Ellen was Mary Ellen. She was just caring. It didn't matter who it was in school. If it was somebody who was supposed to be head of the class, farmers to drug dealers, she spoke to them. They were all her friends." Todd admitted that he and Mary Ellen questioned, "Why us? What did we do to deserve it?" Neither of them could answer those questions. Todd concluded his thoughts about Mary Ellen: "It's like she was still around, and she was like steel. I don't think anything bothered her. You know, she didn't let anybody know that things bothered her. We cried together. She was so special. Some nights I think about why I got it and then I'd think about Mary Ellen, who never did anything wrong. She was always there for you. In school if you needed someone—find Mary Ellen." Todd, at present, considers himself one of the lucky ones since he has been in remission for a few years.

Ellen Z, Mary Ellen's primary care nurse, added her thoughts about Mary Ellen's willingness to help others. "I remember how good she was in talking to other kids who had it. She was always willing to go in and talk and keep a very positive attitude, even though she was sick."

11

❦

AT THE CHECKUP IN NOVEMBER, THE DREADED MONTH, ALL
went well. When Dr. Guinan decided to skip the December checkup and said, "Go home and enjoy the holidays," we were delighted
to have a bit of breather.

The next visit to the Clinic was January 9. Mary Ellen had
planned to fly to Bangor the following day to visit Wendy Cooper.
She was to stay overnight with Shelley and Barnett Goverman,
leaving for Maine in the morning. This Clinic visit revealed evidence of a new tumor in her lungs. It seemed as if all would go
well for a short time period, then Mary Ellen would again metastasize. How we hated those checkups! I know Dr. Guinan felt as we
did. To have to be the constant bearer of bad news must have been
discouraging, especially when we all knew how hard Mary Ellen
fought the disease. She should have been victorious since she
struggled and battled so fiercely.

Again we were faced with the decision, "What to do?" And
again Dr. Guinan had an answer to our question. For this time
there was to be no thoracotomy, but rather a new protocol. There
had been some good luck with a protocol called CHIP, using an
investigational drug to slow the growth of the tumor and to learn
more about the possible side effects of the drug which would be
given during a two-hour infusion in the Clinic. After three weeks
there would be an evaluation, and if the tumor had not gotten any
worse, there would be a second treatment. We knew that each
decision was made with input from many doctors associated with
the Clinic. Therefore, we were aware that the best care possible
would be ours. Again we readied ourselves for chemo treatments.
The possible hair loss and nausea were two disadvantages that
Mary Ellen said she could handle if the drug did its job.

After we made the appointments for our return visit for chemo,
Mary Ellen said, "I don't know if I really want to go to Wendy's."

Although we understood her feelings, I answered her, "You've looked forward to this week since December. Let's call Wendy and explain the situation. Don't say no until you've talked to Wendy."

Wendy assured me, "If Mellon wants to come, we want her to spend the week with us as planned."

Mary Ellen agreed, saying, "I really want to go. I know I'll have a great time with Wendy, Andy, and Smitty, going snowmobiling and all." Putting aside the bad news and the upcoming chemo, she called Wendy to say she'd be there as planned.

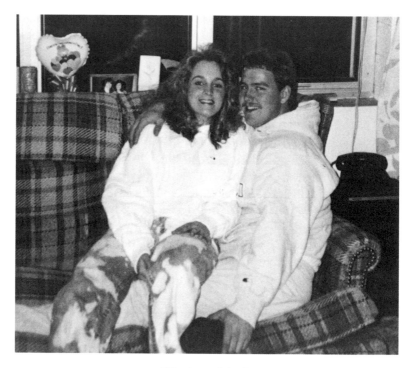

Wendy and Andy

We spent the evening eating Chinese food with Shelley and Barnett. Jimmy and I drove home and Mary Ellen stayed. Shelley reported to us the following day after she had driven Mary Ellen to Logan Airport, that when Mary Ellen saw the little commuter plane destined for Bangor, she became a bit nervous. The week was great, however, and she returned home ready to start the second semester, knowing the CHIP treatment was scheduled for January 20.

On January 20, Jimmy and I picked up Mary Ellen at the college. As usual she was ready, coming out of the dorm with the kids who were going off to their 8 o'clock classes. She yelled her goodbyes, adding, "See you guys on Monday." I couldn't help but think then that life certainly had delivered us a bitter blow. "The amputation was enough," as Jimmy frequently said. How often her life had been interrupted for these chemo treatments! If only we could have hit upon a secret formula. The Ifosfamide seemed to do the trick for at least ten months before a relapse. I marvel at how she kept struggling with all of the possibilities Dr. Guinan could discover. It never occurred to her nor to us to tell Dr. Guinan, "This is it. I don't want to try anymore." We just kept on with the hope and prayer that maybe this time we'd be lucky.

CHIP was administered in the Clinic, taking two or three hours in all. Afterward we planned to go to Margaret Ball's overnight so that if Mary Ellen developed any violent nausea, we'd be near the hospital and could take her for medication. She tolerated the drug fairly well and we were able to return home, letting her rest over the weekend before returning to classes on Monday. Another appointment would be scheduled after two or three weeks, during which there would be the inevitable blood tests.

Life would go along as usual, we hoped, until the blood tests indicated a trip to Boston for an X-ray and, if the tumor showed a good response, another treatment.

With the resuming of chemo treatments and possible hair loss, Mary Ellen became disturbed, since Danielle's wedding was all set for the last week in April.

"I can't be bald for the wedding," she lamented. "But I'm not wearing that wig." It really wasn't too attractive a wig, so we consulted the Clinic staff, who referred us to a wigmaker in Brookline. We planned to make an appointment with her if hair loss seemed to become a problem. In the meantime, we would hold off on the wig for a few weeks to see what transpired.

12

THE FIRST TWO BLOOD TESTS INDICATED THE USUAL LOWER-ing of the white count but everything else seemed okay. As the tests were monitored by Dr. Guinan, and since the results weren't startling, we were just about to plan the next visit when a test on February 3 indicated a very low platelet count. (A low platelet count is serious since the platelets, a main component of the blood, seal up injured areas and prevent hemorrhages.) When I reported the test result to Dr. Guinan, she indicated, "I think we need a platelet infusion." Rather than making the trip to Boston for the transfusion she said, "Check with Dr. Gallup to see if a transfusion could be done at Sharon Hospital."

I immediately called Dr. Gallup who replied, "I'll do all I can but I don't think we'll be able to get blood from Farmington (The University of Connecticut Medical Center) until tomorrow."

Dr. Guinan said it was necessary to transfuse on that day. She didn't want Mary Ellen to wait. Never having experienced a trans-fusion before, we were a little uptight as we tried to get the wheels in motion. In the meantime I called Mary Ellen at school, telling her of the drop in the platelet count and warning her, "Stand by! We may have to make a trip to Boston, but Dr. Gallup and Dr. Guinan are trying to work something out. Go to class if you feel okay and I'll get back to you."

In the meantime, Dr. Gallup and Dr. Guinan decided to try Baystate Medical Center in Springfield, since they both knew Dr. John Kelleher, a pediatric oncologist associated with the hospital. Dr. Gallup called back in a very short time and told us, "It's all set with Baystate. Call Linda, Dr. Kelleher's nurse, to arrange the transfusion. She's expecting your call." How great these doctors were to work so well together, thinking of Mary Ellen all the while and what would be easiest for her! I called Linda, who told us to report before 11 a.m., if possible.

I quickly called Mary Ellen and said, "Be ready by 10:45. Daddy and I will be at school to take you to Baystate." Upon our arrival, Dr. Kelleher and Linda did the preliminaries as the staff prepared for the platelet transfusion. Since this was all new to us, we asked many questions. Everyone was so considerate that we felt at home immediately, as if we were at the Jimmy Fund Clinic since all the procedures were the same. While Mary Ellen had the transfusion, a member of the staff brought us our lunch. This was the beginning of a close relationship between Mary Ellen, Dr. Kelleher, and Linda which enabled us to use Baystate as a backup for Boston. Mary Ellen was indeed lucky, since during the last year of her struggle she often needed medical assistance hurriedly and Dr. Kelleher was always available.

After the transfusion, we drove her back to school and, as she reported to the girls in the dorm, "It was no big deal. I don't feel any different now that the platelet count is up." Dr. Kelleher would monitor the blood counts and send the results to Dr. Guinan. Mary Ellen had three tests scheduled for the 6th, the 9th, and the 11th. In a week's time the counts were fine, and Dr. Guinan was pleased with the platelet count, which was up to 86,000. (A count below 50,000 can prove dangerous.)

13
❧

THE WEEK FOLLOWING THE PLATELET TRANSFUSION, MARY Ellen occasionally experienced shortness of breath, which she attributed to the climbing of several flights of stairs to classes. Her close friends, Amy, Wendy, and Julie, and the other girls in the dorm knew she was experiencing a problem breathing, but they also knew that if Mary Ellen were concerned, she would confide in them.

Later, Julie Gustafson, reflecting upon that day in February, remembered seeing Mary Ellen sitting on one of the benches on the other side of the campus from the dorm. As she spoke with Mary Ellen, who uncharacteristically had little to say, Julie noted on the way back to the dorm that her breathing was quite labored. Everyone in the dorm was concerned and urged Mary Ellen, "Lie down and you'll feel better." "Maybe you just have a little cold." All of the advice was given with concern.

However, Julie remembers Mary Ellen crying, another highly unusual characteristic. Julie told everyone to leave and then said, "Mary Ellen, we're going to the hospital." Julie said that Amy, the usual transporter, wasn't around, so she had to borrow a friend's car. "Off we went to Baystate with me grinding gears all the way."

Once at Baystate, thanks to the previous visit for the platelet transfusion, Dr. Kelleher knew Mary Ellen. He was immediately notified and directed admissions to send her to his office. After a quick check, he sent her to the pediatric unit, much to her dismay since, as she put it, "I am almost twenty-one."

After Julie called us from the hospital, Jimmy picked me up at school and we quickly drove to Baystate, arriving in the middle of the afternoon. X-rays had been done and the culprit was identified as a tumor resting on her left bronchi, causing shortness of breath. Dr. Kelleher had contacted Dr. Guinan and plans were made to transport Mary Ellen the next day to Children's in Boston, with the possibility of radiation treatments to attempt to shrink the tumor.

Later, as Julie and I discussed this ordeal, she mentioned that she and Amy, as they sat in the hospital waiting for us to arrive, talked about the other times Mary Ellen had been hospitalized. "It always seemed like it would be okay. We knew she'd bounce back. Sometimes it was scary and we weren't sure, but the next day there she'd be, back in the dorm. It was just a miracle sometimes when you saw her from one day to the next."

We were as concerned as the girls at this point, but knew that everything that Dr. Guinan could do would be done, so again we put our faith and trust in the Lord. Jimmy and I stayed after the college kids left for the evening and kept Mary Ellen company. She was now using oxygen and was much more comfortable. We called Jim Jr. to tell him what was happening and that we'd be home later in the evening, with the trip to Boston scheduled for the next day. We asked him to call Grandpa, since he always wanted to be informed whenever any new situations arose. I planned to travel with Mary Ellen in the ambulance and Jimmy would meet us at the hospital. We would leave in the early afternoon on February 18, my birthday. Then we called Katherine in Fredericksburg to give her the details of Mary Ellen's latest relapse. She and Mary Ellen chatted while we went to the cafeteria for supper.

The next day, when we arrived at Baystate, Mary Ellen was busy with company from school. As I went to the cafeteria for coffee, a young man wearing a stethoscope said, "Hi." I nodded as I went on my way, thinking he was a friendly young intern or resident. When I returned to Mary Ellen's room, there was the same young man.

Mary Ellen introduced him, "You remember Roland Gelinas, don't you?"

I laughed as I said, "Oh, I thought you were a doctor." Roland wore the stethoscope because he was doing an internship in the cardiac rehabilitation unit through his program at Springfield College. Since that day, he has been Doctor Roland to Jimmy and me.

After lunch, as Mary Ellen bid goodbye to all who came to see her off, we prepared for the ambulance ride. Since neither of us had ever ridden in an ambulance, we were looking forward to the experience. Mary Ellen joked, "If you hang out with me, never a dull moment."

The two EMTs, Bill and Bob, much to her delight, had stocked up on cheese doodles and soda when they heard they had a teenager for a passenger. Mary Ellen was heard to comment about the ride later on, "You might know the better-looking one had to drive!" As we headed toward Boston on the turnpike, Mary Ellen's stretcher faced the back window. Occasionally a car pulled within viewing distance and then she'd wave and smile. The greatest thrill was to go through the toll booth without paying and to hear the siren when a vehicle tended to slow us down.

We arrived at Children's through the Emergency entrance. As

Bill and Bob maneuvered the stretcher through the Emergency Room, Mary Ellen yelled, "Stop!" She had spotted Peggy, one of the nurses who had been at the Jimmy Fund Clinic. She carried on a brief conversation with Peggy as the EMTs waited. Going up in the elevator to our sixth floor, Mary Ellen gave them a running commentary about the hospital and her friends. When we arrived on Division 36, many of our old friends were there to welcome us and to help make Mary Ellen comfortable. It was like old home week—and I'm sure Bill and Bob thought they had indeed transported a celebrity when they viewed our welcome.

The nurses settled Mary Ellen in a private room and called Dr. Guinan. I went downstairs to wait for Jimmy who had left the car at Margaret's and traveled to the hospital by T. Meanwhile, Dr. Guinan came to speak with Mary Ellen and Ellen Z. Since the tumor was in a vital area in her lungs and had grown in size, major decisions had to be made. First and foremost, Dr. Guinan and the radiation staff at the Brigham wanted to try radiation in hopes of reducing the tumor or eliminating it completely. At this point it was imperative that Dr. Guinan explain to Mary Ellen the DNR status. This is the Do Not Resuscitate procedure, whereby a patient in a condition similar to Mary Ellen's is asked to decide whether she wants resuscitation by machines when all else has failed. The machine would not improve the condition, except to make breathing easier. However, speaking and visiting with friends and family would not be possible because the inserted tube would not permit conversation. Mary Ellen indicated she wanted no part of machines.

Later on, Ellen Z remembered this day and the discussion with Dr. Guinan: "The first time I saw Mary Ellen cry since I'd known her was on February 18 as she, Dr. Guinan, and I talked about the DNR. She made the decision to do nothing when and if the planned radiation did not take care of the existing tumor." The decision made, Mary Ellen and Dr. Guinan talked a bit more as plans were discussed for the charting session for radiation the following day. Mary Ellen had made her decision without our being there, but we understood her reasons for being her own person and for deciding her own fate. We hoped and prayed, however, that the radiation would prove effective and that the DNR status would not be necessary.

Another one of her favorite nurses, Kathi Kelly, had the task of transporting Mary Ellen to the Brigham for the charting. Kathy remembers the incident because getting to the Brigham from Children's without going outside, but rather using all of the passageways and elevators, can be puzzling. Kathi said, "I was scared to death because we were all by ourselves and Mary Ellen could hardly breathe. I hoped nothing would happen as we wended our way, not knowing where we were and wondering where we'd come out. As usual, Mary Ellen could joke about the maze of passageways, but I was a bit apprehensive. Eventually we arrived at our destination."

The next day the radiation began. Amy and Julie visited during the first day of treatment. Mary Ellen was still an in-patient and would remain so for a few days. If all went well, and if the tumor showed signs of shrinking, she could go to Margaret's, just reporting to the Brigham twice a day for treatment. As we talked with the girls waiting for Mary Ellen to return from the Brigham, Jimmy and I told them, "Mary Ellen has made the decision not to be resuscitated if this moment does arise. We hope all will go well, but she had to make the decision so the nurses would know how to react if an emergency arose."

Julie later told me, "In our eyes it was saying Mary Ellen realizes that she's only got so much time. And it made us realize that as well." As Julie and I remembered this moment, she continued, "She always bounced back. I never really thought it would be serious. This is the first time that I said she's not going to be around for a long time. It was very upsetting because everyone on campus loved Mary Ellen. Who could help but love that girl? They all knew that Amy and I and Wendy were close to Mary Ellen, all in different ways. Everyone would come up and ask, 'How's Mary Ellen?' After a day of all the same questions I'd answer, 'She'll be back. Don't worry.'"

We all couldn't help but wonder. Would she be back? Could this be the beginning of the end? The end of a valiant struggle? It just didn't seem fair that all she had endured hadn't resulted in a happier ending. Jimmy and I, Katherine and Jim Jr., along with everyone else—family, friends, neighbors, everyone she had come in contact with at Springfield College—lived the next few days waiting for some sign of success with the radiation. We kept asking the nurses and doctors, "Any change yet in the tumor?" Finally after a few days, Mary Ellen could breathe on her own and cautiously Dr. Nancy Tarbell of the radiation unit at the Brigham indicated that we might perhaps experience success. However no final results would be determined until the complete radiation period ended. There would be a total of thirty treatments, twice each day. After a few days, when Mary Ellen showed a positive response to the radiation, she left the hospital and we went to Margaret's. Jimmy and I took turns staying in Boston. He stayed two days and then took the bus home, leaving the car at Margaret's. I came out for the last three days of the week, also by bus, passing, as we said, "on the turnpike." Mary Ellen kept repeating, "Now if I had a car, I could drive myself to the Brigham." Having a car was a sore point, since her sister, Katherine, had bought one while spending the year at home waiting to return to Mary Washington. Mary Ellen kept bugging us to let her buy one so she could go back and forth more readily to school, especially on weekends. She even used Sunday Mass as an argument. Sometimes she missed the Mass on campus and I would become a bit annoyed with her. She'd answer, "Well, if I had a car, I could go anytime off campus."

The radiation definitely did what we all had hoped it would do, and the tumor disappeared. During this time, Dr. Guinan also felt that chemotherapy treatments of VP 16 (a drug that had proved somewhat effective in the treatment of tumors) to be administered in the Clinic could possibly ensure more protection against recurring metastases. Therefore, during the last three or four radiation treatments, Mary Ellen also received the chemo, which fortunately did not make her really ill. Here again we had the expertise of the Dana-Farber organization, trying everything to put a stop to the disease. On March 10, after the last radiation treatment, we left Boston, feeling as if a weight had been lifted. A month before, the outlook certainly hadn't been very bright, but now as we left

Boston, we felt optimistic with the good report.

After Mary Ellen's death, as Julie and I talked about this very grave time in all of our lives, she indicated how the Springfield College community felt as they heard the news of the effect of the radiation on the tumor: "If she got through this, she's going to get through everything. It gave a lot of hope. She's going to lick this." We couldn't help but have the same thoughts. Maybe this was it. This miracle of miracles! The tumor was gone, and perhaps radiation had been the answer.

14
❦

BACK AT SCHOOL, MARY ELLEN BEGAN TO CATCH UP WITH her work. Again the professors, understanding about her days in Boston, gave her extensions on reading assignments and papers. However, as our luck would have it, six days after the last VP-16 treatment and only four days after her return to Springfield, Mary Ellen experienced a bout of nausea that was serious enough for Amy and Julie to take her to the emergency room at Baystate. They called us and we quickly made the trip, arriving about 9 o'clock in the evening. The emergency room was a busy, hectic place, but having an association with Dr. Kelleher made the preliminaries less complicated for the residents on call. Finally, after checking with Dr. Kelleher, they decided to admit Mary Ellen, again to the pediatric unit. She was beginning to be a familiar face to the nurses on the floor.

After trying several drugs to counteract the vomiting, finally they hit upon Decadron, and soon the vomiting ceased. Mary Ellen was discharged after a four-day stay. This time we planned that she should come home for a day or two to avoid any further problems and to be certain she was in good health before returning to the hectic campus life.

When Dr. Kelleher discharged Mary Ellen, he indicated that he and Dr. Guinan had discussed the need for a CT scan of the brain. The reason for this procedure was that the excessive vomiting seemed out of proportion to that usually seen in chemotherapy, and might possibly be evidence of metastases in the brain. Dr. Guinan assured us that this was probably not the case, but the Baystate doctors wanted to be certain. Two days later, before returning to school, Mary Ellen and I reported for the scan. Suddenly our world no longer seemed to be as bright as that day in February when we optimistically left Boston after the successful radiation treatments. Again we were faced with a tremendous ordeal, waiting for a scan and hoping it proved okay. I know Mary Ellen, even though she didn't dwell on the thoughts of a scan, still carried this burden with her, not daring to let herself think of the dire possibilities. Mary Ellen spoke with Danielle to tell her the latest developments, since Danielle and Mike's wedding was fast approaching. How I prayed that nothing would prevent her from taking part in the wedding!

On March 17, Mary Ellen and I arrived for our appointment. While I waited for her, I spoke with Dr. Kelleher and asked him to be certain that no one spoke to Mary Ellen about the results of the scan unless I was present. The one thing I certainly didn't want to happen was the disclosure to her that there were metastases without my being there for support. Dr. Kelleher assured me that he understood and would certainly give both of us the results.

After the scan, we returned to Dr. Kelleher's office. He left immediately to read the scan. In what seemed like an eternity, but was only a few minutes, he returned with the good news. Mary Ellen cried tears of joy as she hugged me and nurse Linda. Dr. Kelleher smiled as he related to our feelings. Another obstacle overturned. Nothing stood in Mary Ellen's path now as she talked about her upcoming trip to Virginia to visit Danielle. Being a "worrywart," as the kids occasionally called me, I mentioned the Virginia trip to Dr. Kelleher. "What if Mary Ellen gets sick while visiting Danielle? What would she do?"

Dr. Kelleher asked, "What's your destination?" When he heard Norfolk, he quickly jotted down the name of a hematologist oncologist associated with a Norfolk hospital. Astounded, Mary Ellen and I asked, "Do you know doctors all over?"

His reply: "We are a select group, so many of us are acquainted."

After this session at Baystate, Mary Ellen returned to school to finish up the week before leaving on spring break and going to Virginia.

Mary Ellen's plans were to fly to Norfolk and spend five or six days visiting and celebrating her twenty-first birthday there. Then Danielle, Mary Ellen, and Danielle's fiance, Mike Lupo, would drive back to Sheffield. We planned a shower for Danielle the Saturday afternoon after their return. What fun it was for me and for all of us to get ready for the shower! Mary Ellen and Katherine also had fittings for their bridesmaids' dresses the morning of the shower. It was a very happy time, as we prepared for the festive days to follow. No thoughts of chemo and all of its side effects crossed our minds while we decorated the living room and dining room with streamers and bells. The shower was a big success and in a way made me a little sad, as I thought of Danielle's being old enough to marry—I still remembered the first days of their friendship when they went to a play group at age four. We had all been through a great deal since then, but we had weathered the storms and now were looking forward to only happy times.

Since the response to the VP-16 had been good, as the X-ray indicated no new growth on the lungs, Dr. Guinan decided to go for another treatment on March 30 and 31. Off we went again to Boston to spend two days, taking the chemo as an outpatient and spending the night at Margaret's apartment. We noticed some hair loss, and since Danielle had given Mary Ellen the ultimatum, "I don't care how much you like wearing bandannas, you're not walking down the aisle in my wedding wearing one," we checked with the wigmaker recommended by the Jimmy Fund staff and found a rather attractive-looking wig. The wig company, run by two very nice women, one of whom wore one of her own products, promised that Mary Ellen would have the wig in time for the wedding.

We still hoped one would not be necessary, but as we all told Mary Ellen, "It's best to be prepared."

When the wig arrived, Mary Ellen put it on, took one quick glance, and proceeded to place the wig in the closet, saying, "It's okay, but I still hope I won't have to wear it. If I have a few strands of hair, I won't wear it." There it sat in the closet, waiting for the wedding day, April 25. As luck would have it, the hair loss was minimal and Mary Ellen was able to get away without wearing it.

15
❦

AFTER THE TREATMENTS, WE RETURNED HOME AND MARY Ellen returned to campus. The necessary blood tests would be done at Baystate, enabling Mary Ellen to remain on campus and to try to catch up with her assignments. On April 12, in the evening, Amy telephoned to tell us that Mary Ellen had been sick all day and wanted to come home. We told Amy, "We'll drive out to get Mary Ellen. It's too late for you to make the trip." Amy insisted she didn't mind the trip to Sheffield.

Later, as Amy and I talked about this particular night, she said, "All day Mary Ellen vomited and we couldn't decide whether I should take her home or to Baystate. She was running a fever and felt awful. It was my Junior Night and I was to go to a party. But I couldn't leave her. As we both lay in the bottom bunk, Mary Ellen with the blue bucket handy, we talked. We were watching the TV show *Family Ties*; the one when Alex's friend died in a car accident. The seriousness of Mary Ellen's illness was becoming more and more obvious. I remember Mary Ellen's comment to me: 'You know, Aim, it really would have been easier if I were hit by a truck.' Then she quickly countered with, 'Just forget that. Forget what I just said. Just take me home.'"

Amy and Mary Ellen arrived home, and as Amy started to leave to return to Springfield, Jimmy and I both said, "Please stay the night, Amy. You can go back early tomorrow morning." I told her,

"It's so late and I'll worry about your driving back alone."

Amy indicated, "I'll be okay and I'll call you when I get back to campus."

We didn't know that this was a special night for her class, Junior Night, and she had planned to attend a party. But this was Amy—completely unselfish when it came to Mary Ellen's welfare.

The following day we returned to Baystate and Dr. Kelleher checked Mary Ellen, only to find she probably had a "bug." He was certain there was no other problem, so we returned home. In a day or two Mary Ellen had recovered. The wedding date was fast approaching, and we all looked forward to this happy event.

April 25 dawned, a day filled with much excitement. Mary Ellen and Katherine looked beautiful; Mary Ellen in a deep-rose-colored gown and Katherine in a lovely mauve. Jimmy, Jim Jr., and I were very proud of them as we took the usual pictures before going to our lovely little white church for the Mass and ceremony. For a year, the wedding had been uppermost in Mary Ellen's mind and heart. She so wanted to be a part of it, but I know she sometimes feared she would not be able to share in this day with Danielle and Mike. I'm also certain that for the entire wedding weekend, with the usual parties, she put aside the thoughts of her next visit to the Clinic scheduled for April 27, two days later. Nothing was going to spoil this weekend—and nothing did.

The following Monday we met Dr. Robert Garcea at the Clinic. He was standing in for Dr. Guinan, who was off on a well-deserved vacation. Mary Ellen had the usual X-ray to determine whether another treatment of VP-16 would be possible. If the X-ray indicated no change since the previous one, then there would be a treatment. However, again we were confronted with the news that there were new metastases in evidence, indicating the VP-16 was not taking hold. Again we had our hopes let down, and again we wondered, "What next?" We felt sorry for Dr. Garcea, who was visibly upset that he had to be the bearer of the bad news. He indicated that Dr. Guinan would return May 1, and that we should make an appointment for that day. We weren't very happy as we left the Clinic to return home and to await the next step in what was appearing to be a one-sided battle. The "Big C," as Mary Ellen called it, seemed to be winning. We may have lost the battle with VP-16, but we hadn't yet lost the war. We would continue to fight because we were certain that Dr. Guinan would have another alternative. We anxiously awaited her return.

Mary Ellen went to campus to resume classes and we came home. The worst part of these Clinic visits, especially after bad news, was reporting the doctors' findings to friends and relatives, especially my parents, who lived every agonizing moment with us. We could count on them to pray for us, and that's what was important now. We couldn't lose our faith nor our hope. We had fought long and hard, and we knew that Mary Ellen would still continue to fight.

16
❦

THE FOLLOWING FRIDAY, MAY 1, WE AGAIN TRAVELED TO Boston, stopping in Springfield to pick up Mary Ellen. We met with Dr. Guinan, who discussed several possibilities for continued treatment. Of course the first possibility, as always, was to do nothing. Dr. Guinan knew that we all felt that all possibilities should be studied and exhausted before we'd succumb to "nothing." We all had decided to keep trying and to keep fighting. Again Dr. Guinan discussed the Ifosfamide treatments that had given some remission previously. She felt Mary Ellen would again meet the criteria for the drug, and since Mary Ellen's earlier response to the drug was excellent, she felt this was the way to go. We agreed, but realizing the problems with the experimental status of the drug and Jimmy's Blue Cross policy's stand on experimental drugs, we knew we would again have to seek aid elsewhere for the hospital costs. And again Massachusetts Electric, Jimmy's employer, came to our aid, indicating that the company would pay for the hospital admissions. There would probably be five hospital stays if the drug proved effective. A creatinine clearance (this test determines whether the kidneys are filtering properly, a necessary criterion before administering the drug since kidney failure is listed as a possible side effect) would be in order to be certain Mary Ellen met the criteria. Therefore, two quarts of urine had to be collected over a 24-hour period. Mary Ellen groaned as she remembered the last time this had to be done. Dr. Guinan advised, "Drink, drink, drink. Anything, even beer!" As we left the Clinic, we collected the two-quart container and headed home. The urine could be delivered to Baystate, where the tests would be done with the results forwarded to Dr. Guinan. We tentatively planned that the first treatment could begin May 8, a week from the visit. Since we had the weekend upcoming, Mary Ellen could fill the container and then return to school on Monday.

The following day, Danielle and Mike arrived home from their honeymoon. Mary Ellen spent most of the weekend out shopping and visiting with Danielle. Sunday evening, when I realized the two-quart container was only half full, and Mary Ellen had been out and about most of the weekend, I'm afraid I lost my temper. Mary Ellen retorted, "If you think I'm going to spend the rest of my life peeing into a jar, you have another guess coming." She really lost control and began sobbing. Then she showed me her arm. "Look," she said, "there's a lump on my arm." And there, above the elbow in the muscle, was a lump that felt as if it might have been a bruise. It moved a bit with the muscle and didn't seem to be attached to the bone.

"Why didn't you tell me when you first noticed it?" I questioned.

She sobbed, "I was afraid. I noticed it before the wedding but I didn't want to ruin the day."

I immediately called Dr. Guinan and related the weekend's situation fully.

First she said, "You can't give up your parenting role."

"I know," I answered, "but it's getting a little more difficult."

About the lump, she indicated I should have Mary Ellen check with Dr. Kelleher the next day to see what he thought. In the meantime, we had to begin again and seriously fill the container so the tests could be made at Baystate and the results sent to

Boston in order to start the Ifosfamide on May 8.

Mary Ellen began to fill the container again, and we talked about the lump. Since there was no pain we felt that was a good sign. We were really grasping at straws, hoping it would not be diagnosed as a tumor. All we could do was wait until Dr. Kelleher checked her arm.

As he checked the lump, Dr. Kelleher felt it wasn't metastases, and again we laughed with joy as we went home with promises of a full two-quart container on the following day. With all of this chemo coming up, Mary Ellen would have difficulty completing the semester. We talked with Cathy Condron, the assistant dean, who assured us she would speak with the professors to see about an extension for three classes. Mary Ellen agreed to work during the summer and to check in with her professors so she could complete all requirements before the fall semester began. That being taken care of, she breathed a sigh of relief as she anxiously awaited the first Ifosfamide treatment. Dr. Guinan had stated previously, "Mary Ellen is at her best when she's on chemo. It's some sort of security blanket for her." And now that Decadron was found to combat the nausea effectively, she wasn't anticipating any vomiting this time. I know Mary Ellen couldn't help but think about the previous Isfosfamide treatments during her year at Berkshire. The drug had given her a ten-month remission. Perhaps again she would experience a remission, enabling her to complete the school year and begin her junior year in September.

The urine tests proved satisfactory, and we planned to report to the Jimmy Fund Clinic on May 9. Dr. Guinan had suggested during the previous visit that a problem might arise regarding the treatment since she had to pull a few strings to have Mary Ellen approved for the protocol. However, she told us, "Don't worry. We'll ask for the protocol on a compassionate basis because Mary Ellen had had such good luck with the previous administering of the drug." Since Ifosfamide was still in the experimental stage, however, Bristol Myers, who controlled the drug, might not release it for administering. In a day or two, Dr. Guinan told us, "They have agreed to the protocol for Mary Ellen." She added, "If they had denied her this chance for a few months' remission, I would have gone to the newspapers."

We, too, agreed that we would also have gone public if the need arose. If this drug could buy Mary Ellen some quality time, then come hell or high water, we'd do everything necessary to make certain she could have the treatments.

Again Dr. Guinan did all humanly possible for Mary Ellen. She fought alongside us and as hard as we did for the same result—at this point, to give Mary Ellen all the time possible. We all knew that the struggle was becoming more and more one-sided as the disease seemed to be edging toward victory, but we would not give up until every avenue had been exhausted.

Mary Ellen spent the next six days on Division 36 receiving the Ifosfamide with the drug Mesna, which was to counteract any damage that might possibly be done to the kidneys by the Ifosfamide. During this hospital stay, the Decadron seemed to control the nausea, so Mary Ellen did not experience the vomiting that usually went with the treatments. She was heard to remark, "Why didn't you guys try Decadron before this? Think of all the pain and strain I'd have been saved if I hadn't puked so much! Oh, well, better late than never!"

Despite the fact that the treatment went better than expected, Mary Ellen returned home a bit down in the dumps. She had missed the final days at school, the exams, the parties, the good-byes. Amy and Julie were to stay on campus for the summer to work. Amy packed up Mary Ellen's belongings, and Jimmy and I drove to the campus one day to collect them. This, too, made Mary Ellen feel bad, since she didn't have the fun of getting all her things together. In September, she and Wendy Cooper planned to room together. Amy would move off campus for a few reasons. She would be doing a great deal of student teaching, for one, and as she confided one day after Mary Ellen's death: "I needed time away from campus and from Mary Ellen. I had to start dealing with all that was happening. I needed to be alone, and the best way to do that was to move off campus. At first Mary Ellen wanted to move with me, but we talked and decided it would be best if she remained on campus. I knew all would be well since she and Wendy had a great friendship, and I knew that Wendy would look after her as I had done."

After this first Ifosfamide treatment, when Mary Ellen returned home from Boston, Tammy Gebo, the physical therapist who had worked with her the preceding summer, made some banana chocolate chip muffins, Mary Ellen's favorite, and rode her bike down to the house. Tammy remembers this visit, saying, "I didn't think anyone was at home so I planned to come in and to leave the muffins. I heard crying and when I looked up, there was Mary Ellen with tears in her eyes. Mrs. Welch told me Mary Ellen wasn't feeling well. I had never seen this side of Mary Ellen's illness. I didn't know what to say, so I hugged her, wiping her tears, and telling her I was sure she'd feel better soon. I rode some twenty-odd miles that afternoon, crying all the way."

17

AFTER THE FIRST CHEMO TREATMENT, THE BLOOD TESTS WERE necessary again. Four days after the treatment, as we arrived for the blood test at Baystate and as Dr. Kelleher checked her over, Mary Ellen admitted that she really didn't feel great. "It's probably a cold," she stated. When nurse Linda took her temperature, which was elevated, and told us the white count was relatively low, Dr. Kelleher determined she should remain in the hospital just to be sure there was no infection. Devastated, Mary Ellen cried. Linda and I talked with her; and I know she realized that hospital-ization was necessary, but she was becoming very tired of all the tests and IVs. It was very difficult now for the technicians to find any veins at all, so putting in an IV was indeed a painful experi-ence. Mary Ellen's veins had virtually collapsed, making the draw-ing of blood even worse. She wanted to be brave and not cry and yell with the pain but the search for good veins was excruciating. We all told her, "If you want to yell, go ahead. We don't blame you."

After she was admitted I returned home, and when Jimmy came home from work, we both returned to Baystate, hoping the doctors would have pinpointed the reason for the fever. The low white count, we knew, was a side effect of the Ifosfamide. We had lived with the low counts, but the fever could prove serious. When we reached the hospital they still weren't certain, as the tests were still in progress. In the meantime, Mary Ellen didn't feel too bad and was able to eat a little and drink her favorite, iced tea. Amy and Julie came to visit. This picked up her spirits a bit. We left with promises to return the next day.

The next day it was decided that due to the infection, she couldn't leave her room. While the counts were low, they wanted to protect her from any more serious problems. As we arrived to spend most of the day with her, she filled us in on her visitors. Our pastor from Sheffield, Father Frederick Heberle, had stopped by, as did our former pastor, Father Francis Sullivan. Ken Childs, the minister from Springfield College, spent some time with her, as did Amy and Julie. When Amy heard about the visitors of the cloth, she retorted, "Okay, I'll send the rabbi tomorrow."

After a few days of confinement, the fever disappeared and Dr. Kelleher indicated we could take Mary Ellen out for a ride, for some ice cream and even for a picnic. During Memorial Day weekend we packed a picnic lunch and Jimmy, Katherine, Mary Ellen, and I went to Forest Park in Springfield for an afternoon outing. This really restored her cheerfulness, and by now she was extremely anxious to leave the hospital scene. After eight days the counts were normal and the fever was gone so the possibility of a very serious illness was again avoided. She came home at the end of May and would have about two weeks before returning to Boston for the second Ifosfamide treatment.

18

WHILE MARY ELLEN WAS UNDERGOING THE CHEMO TREAT-
ments, my parents had returned to their Hillsdale home. My
father had finally consented to the hiring of a nurse, an LPN, to
help my mother with the household duties; Aunt Rita and Aunt
Marian were also staying at the house. We spent a great deal of
time there and noticed that Grandpa wasn't in the best of health.
We encouraged him to go to a local doctor to establish a rapport
so that if he became ill he wouldn't have to make a trip to Scarsdale.
This he finally did, relieving us just a bit.

Before the next Ifosfamide treatment, Dr. Guinan and Mary
Ellen decided to have Dr. Levey implant a central line called a
Hickman, from which blood could be drawn and into which
chemo could be given since this central line was a direct line into
the veins. This meant that there would no longer be the pain
resulting from searching for a vein to support an IV. Twice each
day Mary Ellen had to flush the direct line to the vein and three
times each week she had to replace the small covering of the line.
She had no problem taking care of the line, but upon realizing
that swimming and diving were no longer possible because of the
possibility of infection, she was a bit sad. "I'll miss horsing around
with you guys in Grandpa's pool," she moaned. Our friends the
Sewards had a floating chair they used in their pool and were
more than willing to let Mary Ellen borrow it. She may not have
been able to dive, but she spent many a happy time floating
around the pool in her chair. Needless to say, the technicians and
all the others who had struggled to find veins rejoiced now that
the line was in. Mary Ellen added a rather large red plastic container for the needles used to flush the line with Heparin, as well
as the swabs and bandages to keep the line protected, to her
accoutrements. During this visit to have the line implanted and to
undergo another chemo treatment, Dr. Guinan noted that the
lump on Mary Ellen's arm had become softer and smaller. We

were grateful that the lump had proved to be not so serious a situation.

Before Mary Ellen's Great Barrington therapist, Tammy Gebo, graduated from the University of Connecticut in May, she had to write a paper dealing with an ethical issue in health care. She chose to prepare a questionnaire concerning the objectives of hospice. She asked me if I'd mind completing a questionnaire, and she also sent one to Mary Ellen. This one she immediately regretted. When she called me to ask my advice, I said, "If Mary Ellen feels uncomfortable in answering the questions, she'll let you know."

Mary Ellen returned the completed questionnaire the following week. Tammy shared Mary Ellen's answers, particularly the one dealing with thoughts about death and the meaning of death. Mary Ellen answered Tammy's questions simply and sincerely by writing, "Death to me means peace and a chance to begin a new life with those who have gone before me. I want my parents to take care of me and the arrangements."

Mary Ellen's simple thought about death reflects the religious belief that we taught our children. I'm certain that her peaceful final days were so because of her trust in the Lord and His Blessed Mother. These thoughts she expressed almost a year before her death. I know she had to have seriously reflected on death, since the treatments weren't really taking effect. The miracle about all of this was that she could carry on and never let her spirits show her deepest feelings. How special she was to Our Lord, since He surely helped her cope with this heavy burden!

Early in June Mount Everett graduated the seniors, and Jimmy, Mary Ellen, and I made the rounds of graduation parties, completing the circuit at Bob and Pam Krol's home since their oldest, Joe, was celebrating. Mary Ellen, in a definite party mood, had had a few gin and tonics during the course of our partying. About 10:30 that evening, as the Krol party was beginning to wind down, she turned to Karen Smith, a friend, and exclaimed, "Let's go out to 20 Railroad (a local restaurant and pub) and be bad!" This they did. Luckily we arrived shortly after to find Mary Ellen really ready to call it a night.

Karen remembered a time in April 1988, when a tired Mary Ellen was resting at Kelly Milan's. Karen had just spent three weeks at a drug and alcohol rehab center and she looked forward, perhaps a bit nervously, to beginning life anew. Karen indicated, "I was feeling a bit sorry for myself."

As the three of them visited during the course of the afternoon, and Karen expressed her anxiety, Mary Ellen looked her in the eye directly and said, "Why are you complaining?"

This brief comment, Karen later confided, "Set me straight. I told myself if Mel could continue her fight, there's nothing to stand in my own path, if I really want a life free from addiction." Karen continued, "Seeing Mel, especially when she wore her favorite pink Guess overalls, her very appearance gave me courage. If Mel can strive to live her life to its fullest despite her many physical defeats, I can certainly overcome any obstacles. I owe my steadfastness on the road to sobriety to Mel."

Before the next treatment and after I had finished school, Mary Ellen and I planned a trip to the Lighthouse Inn in West Dennis. We looked forward to lying by the pool and sunning ourselves on the beach. Mary Ellen had to complete the three courses designated by the college before school began in September, so this break was a welcome change before she worked in earnest on these courses.

The end of June found Jimmy and me taking Mary Ellen again to Boston for another round of Ifosfamide and Mesna. The nausea was minimal again, thanks to the Decadron, making the six days in the hospital almost bearable. Mary Ellen was even able to eat Chinese food, compliments of Shelley and Tammy Gebo, as well as pizza, compliments of the nurses. During the Ifosfamide treatment, Tammy visited Mary Ellen while she was undergoing treatment. Tammy tells about this visit, seeing Mary Ellen hooked up to the IV while experiencing the drug: "This was my first encounter with Mary Ellen the cancer patient. She had no hair and wore a pink bandanna. She was hooked up to a machine which monitored her chemo and seemed to ring or beep every time she moved. Mary Ellen was thin and pale. The day before when we ate Chinese, I was fine with her mom's company and

Shelley's, but today I was nervous and apprehensive. I asked Mary Ellen if she wanted to or could go into the courtyard. She indicated she'd like that and asked the nurses to set up the chemo on the wheelchair. As I pushed her, I was nervous because I knew nothing about all this stuff she was hooked to. I was so nervous that when we'd hit a bump, the bottles banged together. I let go of the chair to stop the bottles from hitting each other and the wheelchair rolled forward in the grass, almost knocking Mary Ellen onto her face. She turned to me and said, 'What the *hell* are you trying to do to me? Kill me?' For the moment I felt like the entire hospital was staring at me. Then Mary Ellen started laughing, just a little bit. And then a little bit more. Before long, the two of us were laughing so hard our stomachs hurt. Mary Ellen had this wonderful sense of compassion. She could make anyone feel at ease, just by the way she looked or smiled at you. She could turn a serious situation into a humorous one. She did this as I recall, when she told one of her roommates, a post-op fusion patient, to "resist the tempation to push on your first 'dump,' just sit there and wait for it to fall out."

The treatment completed early in July, we returned home to the preparations for July Fourth at Grandpa's with the usual crowd. My father had experienced some problems walking, but stubbornly he kept telling us he was okay. Bernadette, their nurse, and he were starting to get along since he realized now that her services were invaluable. She kept us informed, so if there were any serious happenings regarding his health, we'd know immediately. Grandpa looked forward to his picnic, the highlight of the summer. We could all invite whomever we wanted, but his guest list was reserved for his very special people. If you received a direct invitation from him, you knew you were special. Charlie "Bub" Reynolds, whom Grandpa had known since he'd bought the house in 1944 and whom Grandpa had watched grow along with the rest of the Reynolds family, was one of Grandpa's special people. Since 1944, most of the Reynolds boys, as well as their father, Ray, had all worked for Grandpa in some capacity. This summer Bernadette confided in me that she had received a verbal invitation from Grandpa and considered herself to be now a very special friend rather than just an employee. The picnic, as usual, was a fun event with Nanny, Grandpa, Aunt Rita, and Aunt Marian getting reacquainted with children, grandchildren, and great-grandchildren.

19
🍎

A WEEK OR TWO AFTER THE HOLIDAY, MARY ELLEN REPORTED again to the Clinic for the third in the series of Ifosfamide. The chest X-ray showed no new growth nor further metastases in the lungs, and for this we were very grateful. The treatment thus far had presented no major problems such as nausea and dehydration, always a possibility when dealing with chemo. The blood tests showed the counts quickly bouncing back after being at the usual low after a treatment. All in all, we were sailing along smoothly, taking one day at a time. Mary Ellen had worked on the assignments for the three classes and was looking forward to returning to campus at the end of August. Katherine was completing her job at the Red Lion Inn and was extremely happy to be returning to Mary Washington College in Virginia, in August after her year's academic probation. Jim Jr. was at the nursery as the assistant manager of the Garden Center, enjoying golf during the summer months, a welcome respite from the rigorous youth hockey coaching schedule during the late fall and winter. On July 10 we all celebrated Mary Ellen's godson Corey's first birthday with a big party at the Milans. There were a few concerts at Saratoga with Tammy Jervas as the summer began to wind down and thoughts turned to school.

Early in August, Aunt Rita frantically called me one morning: "The ambulance has taken your father to the hospital in Great Barrington."

It seems that he had experienced some chest pain in the early morning, and Bernadette decided to call the ambulance. I quickly went to the hospital and found him sitting up in bed reading the newspaper. "Did you need a good rest?" I asked him. He certainly looked great and didn't seem to be any the worse for wear. My brother, Donald, had consulted with the local doctor, who had, in turn, spoken with Dr. Pierson in Scarsdale. It was decided after some tests that the best place to be was the University of Massachusetts Medical Center at Worcester. In a day or two arrangements would be made to transfer him there, under the care of a cardiac specialist for consultation and treatment. We all agreed to this, but our thoughts immediately turned to Nanny, who would certainly need moral support. Along with the aunts, Bernadette was a godsend, especially now. Aunt Ruth and Uncle Frank from Bayside called to say they'd come to stay and do what they could. We breathed a bit easier, knowing that there would be plenty of willing hands to help out. Our schedule, with Mary Ellen due for another treatment August 17 and my driving down to Virginia with Katherine on her way to school on August 18, didn't lend itself to much free time. We certainly were relieved to know that all the family would pitch in and help us out during these few weeks.

20
❧

WHEN WE RETURNED TO THE CLINIC FOR THE NEXT IFOSFAMIDE, Dr. Guinan indicated that there had been a check on Mary Ellen's protocol and it was noted that due to minor bodily deterioration Mary Ellen did not explicitly meet the criteria set forth. Since this drug was experimental, the government kept pretty close scrutiny on those receiving it and there were rigid guidelines to be observed, but Dr. Guinan felt this drug perhaps would be a last chance to slow down the tumor growth. However, because of the deviation from the guidelines, the protocol was changed somewhat, and she now would be on an individualized therapy. The dosage of the drug would not be the established dosage, but rather one compatible with her previous response to the treatment in June. Again Dr. Guinan considered Mary Ellen's desire to continue her battle until such a time when we all might come to realize the war was done.

After Jimmy and I saw Mary Ellen settled, ready to begin the treatment, we planned to return home, stopping at the Worcester Medical Center to visit my father, who was scheduled for a triple bypass operation the following day. I wanted to be with him the next day and suggested I change our plans to go to Virginia for Katherine's return to college. He answered emphatically, "No, don't change your plans. Donald and Lorraine [my brother and his wife] will be here, and I know how much Katherine has looked forward to returning. I'll be fine, and I'll see you when you get back from Virginia."

The day of the operation, August 19, we packed Katherine's car, and she and I got an early start on our way to Virginia. We arrived at my cousin Rita Barringer's late in the afternoon. I had planned to call home to check on my father at 7 p.m. When I finally got through to Jimmy, I heard sobs in the background as Jim Jr. reacted to the news they had just received, that Grandpa had died. I had known there was the possibility of my father's not making it, and I knew from what he had said the day before that he knew, too. I hadn't dwelled on those thoughts as I put my faith in God that all would be well and that the operation would be a success. All I could think about at this moment was the questionnaire he had asked me to help him complete that last time Jimmy and I saw him. To the question "What type of activities do you want to engage in after the surgery?" he replied, "I just want to be able to do some gardening and walking." He loved "puttsing," as he called it, in his garden. In fact, the vegetable garden had, in years past, grown to a small truck farm size. I cried as I remembered this comment. Jim Jr. was so very fond of his grandfather, and for several years he had worked in Hillsdale during school vacations, learning a great deal from him. We were all shocked at the news as I gave the details to Katherine, Rita, and her family. Katherine

160

wanted to drive me back home the next day. "No, Katherine," I answered. "Grandpa knew how much returning to school meant to you and he'd not want you to upset your plans."

It was decided that Rita would see that she got settled in Fredericksburg, and the next morning Katherine would drive me to the airport so I could fly into Hartford, where Jimmy would meet me. As we talked, Rita said to me, "All day I've been thinking about you and Uncle Donald [my father]. Do you remember when my father died?" Of course I remembered. Jim Jr., Mary Ellen and I were visiting Rita's family in the spring about twenty years ago when she received word from her brother in New York that her father had died. Rita and I had been very closely brought up, our mothers being sisters. "How ironic and how fitting that I should be with you when my father died, and you with me."

As I spoke to Jimmy, I cried, "Mary Ellen. We have to tell her, but how?" She and her Grandpa had had such a special relationship. He was so very proud of all of her accomplishments and made it a point to keep all of his friends informed about her doings. She was in the process of the Ifosfamide treatment, but I had to let her know. We entertained the thought of not telling her until it came time to pick her up, probably August 24. "But what if she tried to call him at Worcester, which she might very well do?" I commented. "No, we have to tell her this evening. I'll call her." Jimmy hung up with the agreement that I would call Mary Ellen and then call him back. This would be the most difficult of calls.

I decided to call Ellen Z, hoping she'd be on duty that evening. As luck would have it, she answered the phone at the nurses' station. As I told her, I asked about Mary Ellen. "She's fine," said Ellen. "In fact, she has company now. Some friends from school are here. She's doing real well, no vomiting, and she's in good spirits." Ellen and I decided that she'd walk down to Mary Ellen's room, and in a minute or two I'd call Mary Ellen. At least she'd have Ellen's support. The nurses loved her and I knew they'd be there for her.

I dialed her room and as she answered her phone, so upbeat, my heart sank. After a few comments about our trip, Katherine, and Rita's family, I said, "Mary Ellen, Grandpa's operation wasn't

161

a success and he died this evening. I'm so sorry to have to give you this bad news." She cried, as did I. "Oh, why did he have to do that?" she sobbed. "How could he do this to me?"

Ellen took the phone. "Don't worry, Mrs. Welch. We're all here for Mary Ellen. We'll take care of her." Life without Grandpa would be empty indeed. I could only hope that we would all now have a voice close to God, His Son, and our Blessed Lady to intercede for us.

I realized the next few days would be difficult, to say the least. Rita's daughter, Anne, called about a plane ticket for the next day as I made my plans to fly home.

21

❦

I ARRIVED HOME TO A VERY SAD HOUSEHOLD. JIM JR. LOVED his Grandpa dearly as did we all. He was visibly upset as he greeted me. I drove to Hillsdale to visit with Nanny. Her reaction was a bit strange. She was naturally devastated, since she and Grandpa had been inseparable, especially since his retirement from Kidder Peabody. It seemed, however, as if she didn't want to talk about his death. The aunts were all there, as was Bernadette. We made our plans to drive to Scarsdale on Sunday to get ready for the two days of calling hours and then the funeral. During these days, Bernadette was indeed a gift from above as she took such good care of our mother. She said to me, as I thanked her probably for the twentieth time, "I loved your father and promised him I'd take care of your mother." Everyone loved our father. One couldn't help but not. He was generous, kind, considerate, and very honest. The many letters from business associates gave us indeed a feeling of pride, since they all praised his sense of honesty and fairness. He would be sorely missed by us, as well as his friends and business acquaintances.

The day before the funeral, Jimmy drove to Boston to get Mary Ellen since she had finished the chemo treatment. They would come directly to Scarsdale. Tammy Gebo told me about visiting Mary Ellen the day after Grandpa had died. Mary Ellen called Tammy the evening after his death. When Tammy arrived at the hospital, she said, "Mary Ellen was different. She asked people to leave the room; she appeared angry and barely spoke to me during the two hours I was there. I finally asked her what was wrong. Mary Ellen, crying, told me, 'My grandpa died yesterday. My mother had to drive Katherine back to school and I needed someone.'" Tammy said, "We both cried. I knew what he meant to her and losing him was like losing a part of herself."

Grandpa was such an important part of Mary Ellen's life. She would truly miss him and especially the fun times at Hillsdale when he'd come down to the pool, see us lying there, and say, "Pretty soft!" He was happiest in Hillsdale and loved our managing to spend so much time there. Mary Ellen spoke with Aunt Rita upon arrival in Scarsdale, saying she couldn't go to the funeral home that evening for the calling hours. Then she simply added, "I'm next." As the cancer seemed to be getting the upper hand, I'm sure Mary Ellen wrestled with thoughts of death and dying.

After the funeral we all returned to Hillsdale, even my mother, since she said, "That's what your father would want me to do." Hillsdale wasn't her favorite place, and my father often kidded about the future of the house after he died. He made certain that were he to die before our mother, she wouldn't be able to sell it. He left the house to us, his children. Again Bernadette and the aunts were with us, looking after things in Hillsdale, as we hired another nurse to assist Bernadette.

22

AFTER THE AUGUST TREATMENT WE FINALLY RECEIVED SOME good news: the lump on Mary Ellen's arm had disappeared. It had been so long since we had had a good report, but now maybe the "old friend" Ifosfamide would do the trick. Of course hair loss occurred, but by this, the third time, Mary Ellen was accustomed to the bandannas and so was everyone else. She returned to Springfield to begin the junior year, having completed the necessary assignments during the summer, receiving nine credits. She was just a bit shy of enough credits to be a full-fledged junior, but we said, "So what? Who cares if it takes a bit more than four years?"

The last Sunday in August, Mary Ellen and I loaded the car and off we went to Springfield. Jimmy and Jim Jr. were playing in a golf tournament, so I had the happy chore of getting her settled. Mary Ellen's wardrobe, known throughout the campus as rather extensive, what with her thirty or forty sweaters and thirty pairs of pants, took up most of the trunk and the back seat. We could have used a U-Haul. Jimmy was, I'm certain, glad that he had a golf game. Luckily, we found a parking place right near the dorm. As we struggled with the hangers, boxes, books, and the rest of her paraphernalia, some guys came by.

"Can we help?" they asked.

"You sure can!" we answered.

Then they looked at Mary Ellen and in unison said, "You look a heck of a lot better than you did last May."

She was tan and had put on a bit of weight and really did look great. How happy she was to be back in the swing of college activity! She couldn't wait to see Wendy and Andy and all the rest of her friends. The arrival was a much happier scene than her departure had been in May. Maybe now the treatments would kill those tumors and let her have a great year. This was our prayer. She had earned a respite from all the pain and tension of treatments. There would be just one more treatment of Ifosfamide in

September, resulting in her missing only one more week of classes. Since the treatments, with the help of Decadron, hadn't made her too sick, she could do reading assignments while in the hospital. And again, the professors were very understanding.

23
❧

DURING THE MONTH OF SEPTEMBER, MY MOTHER EXPERIENCED many problems because of her arthritis and also because of the absence of my father. Even though she rarely talked about him, we knew the pain of her loss was almost too difficult to bear. We felt that she really had lost her will to live. She, too, had fought a battle with a disease, rheumatoid arthritis, since 1948 and now was really tired of all the treatments and medications she had been subjected to all these years. The disease finally took its toll, and my mother died October 6, just 48 days after my father. We again spent the few days preparing for the funeral in Scarsdale. Once more Mary Ellen, along with the rest of our family, faced the death of a close family member. We were happy, however, that our mother's suffering was over and that she again was reunited with our father for eternity. I cannot comprehend how we all would have coped with these two deaths if we had not had our strong religious convictions. We would dearly miss our parents, but we knew they went to a happier existence than we could ever imagine as mere mortals, an existence filled completely with the honor and glory of God, where there would never be pain nor anguish and where they would share their happiness together. Here on earth we suffered because of our loss, but we rejoiced in their togetherness.

24

MARY ELLEN, HAVING PLANNED TO SPEND THE COLUMBUS holiday weekend visiting Danielle and Mike in Norfolk, flew to Baltimore, where she met Steven, Danielle's brother. They did some sightseeing in Washington and then drove to Norfolk. Mary Ellen flew home after a short visit and then back to campus. On October 23 we returned to the Jimmy Fund Clinic for a checkup and to determine if the Ifosfamide had been effective. At this time, Dr. Guinan's notes gave insight into the steps to be taken from this point on in our battle.

> *Mary Ellen comes in today for a routine visit. She is feeling and doing extremely well. She has no pulmonary, bony, or extremity complaints. During the past two weeks, Mary Ellen and I have had an extensive number of conversations about the course of her illness. We have discussed the option of continuing Ifosfamide at this time vs. discontinuing it. A review of her course shows that she had all of her X-ray resolution at the end of two courses and that she has received three courses of Ifosfamide to consolidate those changes. Chest X-ray today was obtained, which again shows no evidence of disease regrowth and shows small scars from the pulmonary nodules, as well as the large calcified mass in the right upper lobe. Because of her desire to continue to participate fully in school, as well as lack of evidence that we are achieving anything further with therapy, we will stop her Ifosfamide at this point and continue to monitor her closely. This course was discussed with parents and the patient again in detail, who agreed that this was the most reasonable course at this point for her, vis-à-vis life-style and her medical care. As well, we discussed the fact that CT scan would not be particularly useful at this point and that we would follow her progression with chest X-rays.*

Over the years, Dr. Guinan and Mary Ellen had developed a close relationship, Mary Ellen feeling extremely comfortable with her, able to discuss boyfriends as well as cancer. We felt indeed fortunate to have such a dedicated woman in charge. We left the

Clinic that day knowing the Ifosfamide had at least stopped any growth and that no new metastases were evident. We could only pray that the drug would again give Mary Ellen the remission she had enjoyed when she first received the Ifosfamide while at Berkshire School. Of all the patients with osteogenic sarcoma known to Children's Hospital staff, Mary Ellen evidently seemed to enjoy the best luck when it came to Ifosfamide.

Since the semester thus far had progressed well, Mary Ellen expected to complete the term with at least a 2.5 GPA. She was very much encouraged with the way her courses were going and thoroughly enjoyed her classes. Several of her friends in the rehab program used her experience with chemo and her own rehabilitation as subjects for papers. Mary Ellen was heard to comment when asked if she again would be a willing subject. "I should get a percentage of all the A's you guys have gotten because of me."

Julie Gustafson remembered the semester and Mary Ellen's really upbeat attitude: "I was living off campus but ran into Mary Ellen early in the semester. We made plans for her to come to dinner and to see the house. When you live off campus, you're kind of hot stuff. Staci and I went by the dorm to pick her up one early evening in Staci's bomb of a car that made an awful racket. I can still see Mary Ellen coming bombing out of the dorm, laughing at the car and at us. We had a great dinner and a lot of laughs. She went to a lot of parties that semester."

Amy, who now lived off campus and was busy with student teaching, and Mary Ellen saw one another occasionally since they did keep in touch, going to lunch or dinner. I'm sure Mary Ellen missed Amy but knew that if she needed her, Amy would be there. Mary Ellen, for the third year, enjoyed dorm life in Abbey with Wendy again as her roommate. Meeting the new dorm freshmen at a get-together made for a rather hilarious experience when Wendy picked up Mary Ellen's prosthesis and shouted, "This is Oliver. If you see him running down the hall, just bring him back and we'll put him in the closet."

The new freshmen, according to Wendy, thought she was a bitch, so cruel, until they saw Mary Ellen doubled up, laughing. Mary Ellen liked the way Wendy teased her. Oftentimes as they walked on campus and the younger students—the "'Shmen"—would say "Hi!," Mary Ellen was bothered by the individual attention. Wendy continued, "People knew me because of her. It seemed that I was Mary Ellen's roommate and I didn't even have a name." Wendy also said, "It bothered her that they'd run and hold the door for her." Eventually, however, as the semester progressed, the "'Shmen" learned to treat Mary Ellen like everyone else. In fact, many students, those who didn't live in her dorm or weren't in her classes, had no idea that Oliver existed.

Amy Watson, a classmate who also lived in Abbey dorm, remembered Halloween during this semester, when they were all preparing for a costume party. According to Amy, "We were all discussing our costumes while Mary Ellen seemed a bit 'down' since she had no idea for a hidden identity. Suddenly I came up with the pirate idea. She loved it! What with her lack of leg and her bandanna since her hair was still not totally grown back, I told her she'd be a great pirate! She agreed and we had a blast at the party!"

The handicap plate on the car continued to bother her and once she asked her father to get rid of it. When Jimmy checked with the insurance people, they indicated that if we were to do so, it might be very difficult to get one later. So we ignored the plate, parking in a regular place rather than the handicap one. Jeanette Cooper remembered meeting Mary Ellen one day in a supermarket parking lot in Great Barrington. Mary Ellen had parked and noted a man, obviously in good shape physically, parking his car in the handicap area. She approached him, drew herself up to her 5 feet 7 inches, and said, "Are you handicapped?" The person indicated he was not. Mary Ellen continued, "Well, you parked in the handicapped area. I have a handicap plate and didn't park there. Look." She pulled up her pants' leg and then trotted off to the store, leaving the man staring after her.

Another instance illustrating Mary Ellen's attitude toward those not so fortunate as she occurred while she was on chemo. A multi-handicapped young lady was moved into her room. The nurses indicated, "Her former roommate couldn't stand the sight of this unfortunate person, so the parents asked that the patient be moved. We knew that Mary Ellen would welcome her." And welcome her Mary Ellen did. If the chemo didn't make her too nauseous, she related to all of her roommates. She had been such a constant visitor to Division 36 that she often acted the part of tour guide.

25
❦

In November we returned for the monthly check-up, remembering that Novembers were usually "bad" months, many little tumors having been picked up during November visits. Mary Ellen was feeling great, but we were apprehensive. Dr. Guinan told us that the X-ray was a bit difficult to read due to all the scarring in the lungs from previous operations, but there didn't seem to be evidence of new tumors. We were delighted and were even more so when she said, "I think we can wait until January for our next visit." It was already November 20 and with the holidays approaching, Dr. Guinan felt that a January appointment would be fine. We left Boston, lighthearted and unconcerned, stopping at Legal Sea Foods for lunch. We took Mary Ellen back to school, with instructions to pick her up the following Wednesday before the Thanksgiving holidays.

We again spent the holidays with my sister Dolores, but this year we were saddened since it was the first holiday without Nanny and Grandpa. Their presence was sorely missed as we reminisced about events that had occurred during the many Thanksgiving holidays spent together. We remembered the comment Grandpa always made after dessert: "Where are the pink peppermints?" Dolores always had a dish of candies for him with his favorite, the pink ones.

Katherine came home for the holidays, and things seemed to be going well for her at MWC. She was working hard and enjoyed being back with her friends. Jim Jr. was involved in the Sheffield

Youth Hockey League, coaching again with Joe Milan. He was also busy with his position at the nursery. As a family we had a lot to be thankful for this holiday, now that all seemed to be moving along smoothly. We could only hope and pray that perhaps now the cancer would retreat a bit, giving Mary Ellen a well-deserved respite from treatments.

Between the Thanksgiving holidays and Christmas, Mary Ellen worked hard at school, completing the semester with no more setbacks. She hadn't done too much skiing the previous season, but now she really felt so good that she wanted to resume the sport. She and Amy went to Vermont one Saturday in December. Amy remembered the day as she wrote about their adventures:

> *I recall the ridiculous Mellon that day, slipping off her friend Oliver and strapping herself to her ski. Mary Ellen was graceful as she paralleled the mountain (as I unathletically followed). We made our way down under the ski lift as skiers on the chairs turned their heads to stare at Mellon—the most incredible sight around (which she was aware of). Suddenly Mellon did one of those fancy, one-legged ski stops. She then waved at the onlookers and pleasantly screamed, 'Hi, guys! Meet you down at the bottom for photos and autographs!' She glided the rest of the way down as I fell and laughed in the snow.*

She was happiest as she navigated the mountain. To ski again, to be free of care and worry, to savor the adulation of the other skiers, to toss aside for a short while the cares and worries of the "Big C," meant everything to Mary Ellen. Being an excellent skier, she indeed attracted the attention of others on the slopes. Whoever observed her could not help but toss aside their own complaints, major or minor ones, as they observed a valuable lesson in courage, determination, and perseverance.

During the holiday season, Mary Ellen also went to Bousquet to ski with Tammy Jervas, whose father owns the ski area. They skied several times and each time Mary Ellen would be heard to say, "Next time I ski without the outriggers and only use the poles." Using the poles would put a tremendous strain on her "good" leg, but since she was obviously in good shape, it was just a matter of time, what with Tammy's egging her on. Using them was like

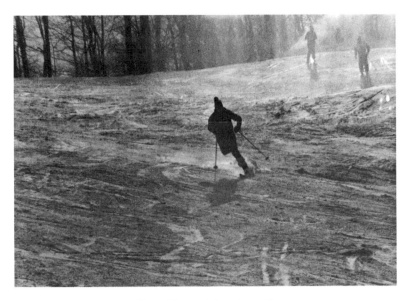

Mary Ellen skiing with poles at Bousquet

climbing a mountain might be for someone else, because she would be putting aside the handicap equipment, proving (mainly to herself) that she had the stamina to "go for it."

Late one afternoon she arrived home, excited and out of breath. "I did it," she yelled as she came in the door with Tammy close behind. Sure enough, she had borrowed a set of poles and accomplished what she had been promising herself she'd do. She was very proud of herself, even though she paid for the adventure the next day when she experienced some pain along her left side where she had had a major incision from a thoracotomy. "It's worth the pain," she remarked.

Even before she fell victim to cancer, Mary Ellen had been one to push herself regarding skiing, softball, and field hockey. She loved these sports and spared nothing when it came to performing. When she lost her leg, she did not lose her determination, perseverance, and love of participation. Despite the prosthesis, she did her best. Jeanette Cooper remembered, when seeing Mary Ellen actively involved at Berkshire, a comment one of her own college professors had made back in 1969-70. Jeanette said, "The professor wrote two words on the board—Ability and Disability—and then explained, "It's ability, not disability, that counts.'"

Jeanette continued, "I think that's exactly Mary Ellen. Even though the leg is gone, I'm still able; I'm not disabled. I'm going through life; here's what I can do. I'm going to do them and I did." Field hockey had to take a back seat, but her stick remained in the closet, a happy reminder of field hockey days at Mount Everett.

Throughout the whole ordeal, her determination and stubbornness became a plus for her. She set herself objectives, which she then proceeded to accomplish. Mary Ellen had little use for whiners and complainers. During a softball game while a student at Mount Everett, her friend Lisa Gulotta was dejected because she thought she wasn't performing well enough on the field. Mary Ellen, ready to pitch, yelled to Lisa, "I'm not throwing this ball until you pick up your head and look alive!" When Mary Ellen couldn't play, she was the strongest fan on the bench, constantly yelling encouragement.

Watching her struggle and fight the disease every inch of the way, I often had to bite my tongue not to become angry with the young people I'd observe at school who I felt were wasting their lives and their talents. Often I'd find myself resenting these students as I thought about Mary Ellen fighting to live and giving it her all. I thought about how great a rehab counselor she would have been had she been given the chance. Later on after her death, Ray Chamberland, our Mount Everett principal, commented as we reflected together on Mary Ellen's twenty-two years on this earth: "We'll never know in our lifetime how many people she influenced or helped."

And that is the crux of the matter. We don't know how long our time on this earth will be; whether it be twenty-two years or sixty-two years. We all have a reason for being and Mary Ellen's reasons must have been to set examples of courage, strength, and determintaion.

The holiday season passed, and Katherine returned to MWC. She and her friend Jennifer talked during the holidays of spending the summer in Georgetown, getting jobs waiting on tables. They were pretty certain of a place to stay, since they knew some girls from MWC who would sublet them a condo in Georgetown. Mary Ellen's plans for the summer were indefinite. However, during spring break in March, she and Tammy Jervas planned to go to Tahoe to do some skiing and then to San Francisco to spend a few days with their skiing buddy and good friend, Artie Hebert, who was attending law school in San Francisco.

Part 5

1
❦

ON JANUARY 8 WE HAD OUR NEXT APPOINTMENT WITH DR. Guinan for the inevitable X-ray and blood work. Mary Ellen was feeling great and had spent a busy vacation skiing. Her hair was also beginning to grow back. It was with the usual trepidation, however, that we awaited the results. The news wasn't good. Dr. Guinan told us, "The X-ray shows increasing disease in the right lung." However, other than a minor pain at times on her left side from the last thoracotomy, Mary Ellen experienced no discomfort. Again we were faced with major disappointment. It seemed as if now each visit brought bad news, as the good news became more and more infrequent. Dr. Tarbell and Dr. Guinan discussed the possibility of radiation therapy. They decided to begin therapy January 14. Since the last radiation treatments in February 1987, had proved successful, we had hopes for some success this time.

As second semester began with the cloud of radiation treatments hanging over her head, Mary Ellen began classes knowing she would have to interrupt them for three weeks. Amy recalls their going out to dinner to celebrate her birthday. Their being alone for a change was a welcome treat, as they had not had much time together during this, Amy's senior year. As Amy recalls, "We were separated this year, but now just the two of us enjoyed one another's company."

Mary Ellen told her, "Amy, I'm really scared about dying. I don't know how to do this gracefully."

Amy replied, "Just do what you do on the slopes. Do what you have to do. You'll know what to do." In remembering this evening, Amy said, "We didn't see each other as much. I needed to separate myself because I'm just so sensitive. I was too involved."

This conversation with Amy was the first truly serious discussion Mary Ellen had with her two closest friends at Springfield, Amy and Wendy. Later in the semester, she and Wendy talked at length about death and dying, and I think it was then that she resolved the process as she came to terms with the realization that death was quite imminent.

Mary Ellen had signed up for eighteen credits, six courses, which I felt was a rather heavy course load. As she said, "If I find I can't handle all of them, I can always drop one or two, since I really only need twelve credits to remain a full-time student."

When the date to begin radiation came, we arranged our schedules so that Jimmy spent two days and I three days each week staying at Margaret's. We reported to the Brigham twice a day: at 7 a.m. and again at 2 p.m. Again, there would be thirty treatments, finishing February 10.

While we were staying at Margaret's, Boston had quite a snowstorm. Having to park the car behind Margaret's apartment house meant shoveling to get the car out for the twice daily trips to the Brigham. I hadn't shoveled snow in years, but the morning after the storm, Margaret and I joined the neighbors as we shoveled out our cars. Mary Ellen came out with us to "direct." As I shoveled, I complained to her and Margaret, "You might know that it would snow during my time here rather than Jimmy's. He's so much better at shoveling than I am."

Despite the storm, we made it to the hospital for the afternoon appointment. Returning to the apartment, we enjoyed a quiet afternoon, when about 4 o'clock Margaret announced, "We had better go outside and shovel again. The snow has stopped and you'll want to be able to get out easily tomorrow morning."

So out we went to clean out the parking area. Mary Ellen didn't join us. "I'll let you guys do it alone this time," she retorted.

One morning in early February at the close of the radiation treatments, Shelley and Mary Ellen took off for a day's skiing trip at Mt. Wachusett, near Worcester. They had a wonderful day, and Mary Ellen said she felt great. Remembering this day, Shelley said, "Mary Ellen would matter-of-factly tell people she was in Boston getting radiation, and she usually skied in the Berkshires. She had a great many admirers! She seemed to feel great, ate a hearty lunch, and skied amazingly well without fatiguing." Other than a scratchy throat due to the radiation, she experienced no side effects. After the treatments, she returned to the Springfield campus and picked up her life again.

On February 28 we returned to the Clinic for the usual monthly check and also to the Brigham for a visit with Dr. Tarbell. Mary Ellen had been experiencing some pain in the lower left lung area where she had had surgery. She attributed the pain to a fall or two taken during the last skiing adventure. With the visit came the report that there appeared to be a regrowth of disease in the left chest wall. Dr. Guinan and Dr. Tarbell both indicated that no further radiation could be done to this area since the disease was so close to the spinal cord. Perhaps surgery could be performed to remove the metastases. Dr. Guinan wanted to talk with Dr. Levey after he had studied the latest X-ray. We would await the decision concerning surgery. In the meantime, Mary Ellen had planned to leave later that day for a ski weekend with her friend Colleen Hax and Colleen's family. On March 19 she and Tammy Jervas planned to go to Tahoe and then to San Francisco. Therefore, Mary Ellen noted, "Any surgery or any more treatments will have to wait until after spring break. I'm not giving up my trip."

Dr. Guinan, who consistently wanted Mary Ellen to do whatever it was that was important to her, whether it be school or trips, agreed that these activities were of the utmost importance and all decisions would be put on hold until later. Besides the recurrence of the disease in the lung, the lump that she had experienced in her left arm almost a year ago had returned. This lump was still a mystery, but Dr. Guinan indicated that it, too, would be watched and a decision reached when Mary Ellen returned to the Clinic in April.

On the return trip to Springfield, where Mary Ellen planned to meet Colleen and then leave for Vermont, we talked very little about the discussions with the doctors. It seemed as if our options were dwindling and that there was little else the doctors could do to combat the disease, which now seemed to be racing toward victory. We did, however, hold on to the hope that a miracle could still happen.

We arrived on campus early in the afternoon after this last terrible Clinic visit, in time for the girls to load up their gear and to head off to the slopes. Colleen lived in Abbey dorm, on the same floor as Mary Ellen and Wendy. She and Mary Ellen shared some good times sitting on her couch, watching the people pass by the window, going to soccer games, Friendly's, parties, and yes, even to the library. Colleen remembers the ski weekend as she writes:

> One of the most memorable times I spent with Mellon was when we went to Vermont, skiing with my family. We left on a Friday, the same Friday she had gone to Boston and returned with some depressing news, but you wouldn't have known it the way she acted—and we laughed so much that weekend.
>
> On Saturday we went skiing with my dad, my brother, and one of his friends. We skied all day and even took videos. Mellon was an amazing skier and skied even the most difficult trails. If someone complained about something that weekend, she would just look at them and with a grin say, "Go big or go home!"
>
> One of the funniest things that weekend happened when we went snowmobiling on Sunday. She and I got on the snowmobile, but we were having a little trouble because her leg kept slipping off the side of it. So Mellon got off, said she'd be right back, and went into the house. When she came back, she had taken off her leg. She smiled as she came out the door on her crutches and said with a laugh, 'That's something you guys can't do!' Then she hopped on the snowmobile and off we went.

2
❦

SINCE DR. GUINAN HAD SPOKEN TO MARY ELLEN DURING THE February visit about the advancing of the disease and the lack of positive response from all of the treatments, Mary Ellen knew now that her time on this earth was more limited than ever. She was very fortunate to have Wendy Cooper for a friend and room-mate, since she and Wendy talked about her condition quite openly and freely. For this reason, she never seemed to want or need to talk with us, her family. I believe she wanted to protect us from the sorrow to come, as she confided in Wendy at this crucial time. Wendy remembered Mary Ellen's words in the early months of 1988: "I know I'm not on death's doorstep, because I know I'm not right there, but I know I'm going to die. I just don't know when. I don't know how soon." Mary Ellen continued, "The last thing I want to do, if there's one thing I want to do, it is to see you and Andy when you get married." This didn't happen, but Mary Ellen was happy to see Wendy and Andy together just a few hours before her death.

Mary Ellen also shared her thoughts about boyfriends with Wendy, since she felt as if she had missed out by not having had a real male-female relationship. Mary Ellen had many boyfriends but not one special one. She questioned this with Wendy: "Why can't someone like me for who I am?"

Wendy reassured Mary Ellen, "I wouldn't let it bother you. College guys are so immature. You know they want one thing. They don't see, they can't see past your having cancer. Or that you have a prosthesis. You don't want anyone on this campus. You'll find somebody." Wendy continued, "Mellon really wondered about sex. I think she felt cheated."

Mary Ellen said to Wendy, "I'm never going to be able to experience that. I'll never be able to have kids."

As Mary Ellen and Wendy continued their discussion about death, its reality, its mystery, she told Wendy, "It had better be the way my mother has described," adding, "At least I'll see my Nanny and Grandpa again."

Wendy indicated that through those early months of 1988, Mary Ellen struggled with the idea of death and dying. But then, as she sorted out the process of living and dying, she seemed to become comfortable with it, even though it seemed she did not wish to discuss it with her family. At one point she confided in Wendy, "You guys have to worry about what you're going to wear in the morning, and I have to worry about whether I am going to wake up or whether I have already died."

When I asked Wendy if Mary Ellen had ever thought she had gotten a raw deal, Wendy answered, "I'm sure she did think that, but she worked it through and came to the conclusion she was needed for some reason." Wendy added what we all knew from the start of this struggle: "She was probably the one in a million that could handle it." Wendy continued, "And she thought that you, her parents and her family, Jim and Katherine, were four in a million to have supported her as you did all along. Katherine, especially, she grew closer to as the two of them talked on the phone often and at length. In one respect, I think she was envious of Katherine; like, why me and not her? And then she was thankful it was her and not Katherine." Wendy concluded with, "Once she said it might have been easier if she had been hit by a truck, gone. But then she reconsidered, saying she wouldn't have been so lucky as to have had those five years to live life to its fullest."

3
❦

DURING THE FIRST WEEK IN MARCH, MARY ELLEN DEVELOPED a cough and a cold. She went to classes but didn't seem to have very much energy. Knowing that her trip with Tammy was fast approaching, she decided to spend some time at home to try to recuperate. Dr. Kelleher prescribed antibiotics, and we hoped Mary Ellen would recover in time for the trip. We had talked with Dr. Guinan, who indicated that Dr. Levey would not be able to remove the new tumor surgically because of its location. She told us that after spring break, however, we would talk about a new chemo treatment. In the meantime, Mary Ellen and Tammy kept in constant touch with one another, Mary Ellen reassuring her, "I'm going with you. I know I'll be okay for the trip." Besides the cough, Mary Ellen's appetite had noticeably diminished. We tried to fix all of her favorites so she'd eat enough to get back her energy.

Both Jimmy and I were really concerned, as she certainly didn't seem to be able to throw off this latest bug as quickly as we had hoped. March 19th was fast approaching. If she did become ill while in San Francisco or Tahoe, Dr. Guinan assured Mary Ellen that she was only a phone call away. This fact eased our minds a bit, as did the fact she would be with Tammy, a very responsible young adult. We spoke with Tammy a few days before the trip, since Jimmy and I felt we should be open about the progression of the disease, which I'm certain Tammy was already well aware of. When I said to Tammy, "Mary Ellen isn't really feeling up to par, and we think you should know that a problem could arise."

Tammy simply commented, "I've been in on this since the beginning. I know. Don't worry."

Before the trip, Mary Ellen spoke with the dean of students and asked to drop two courses, since she now felt she could no longer handle her heavy course load. Dean Condron agreed to the fewer courses. This uplifted Mary Ellen's spirits as she commented, "There's always summer school."

On March 19, Jimmy and I drove the girls to Bradley Airport. What with the skis, poles, outriggers, crutches, and suitcases, they had more than enough to handle. We stopped for a sandwich at the airport and noted that Mary Ellen really didn't feel much like eating. My heart was heavy as I watched her. She wanted so badly to feel great, but in reality she felt sort of "down." This trip had been uppermost in her thoughts since the planning stages many months before, and now it was almost a chore to go through the process of getting ready to board the plane. How badly I wanted to cry for her; to try to make everything all right for her; to ensure a marvelous trip! As departure time grew near, the thrill of the trip and Tammy's spirit caught hold and she seemed to regain a bit of her usual pep.

As they boarded the plane, Jimmy and I couldn't help but wonder what would happen this week. We sincerely prayed that she and Tammy would have a great time with nothing to ruin their vacation, and we thanked God for Tammy, who would take care of Mary Ellen.

Tammy and I talked about this "dream" vacation and the great desire Mary Ellen had to see California and to visit Artie Hebert. As they settled on the plane, Mary Ellen questioned Tammy, "Did my parents give you the third degree about watching over me?"

Tammy replied, "No, they didn't say anything but to have a good time."

Tammy told me, "I think Mel was a bit surprised that you hadn't given me a list of do's and don'ts for taking care of her. She was obviously very happy and felt good that you sent her off without a warning to me. I think her initial reaction was one of surprise as she relaxed, anticipating the trip."

Tammy continued, "When we arrived, I stepped back as Artie

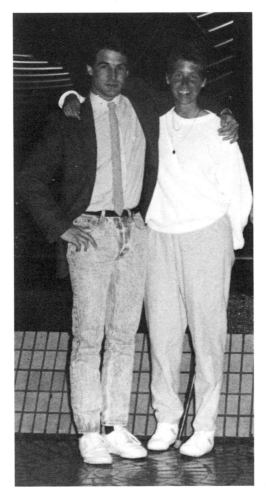

Artie and Mary Ellen

came to greet us. Mel was so excited that she was finally there—the dream come true—as Artie gave her a big hug; he was great. At this climactic moment, she realized her dream but was almost afraid to be too happy in case something dreadful regarding the disease were to happen. She was almost afraid to relax and to enjoy the moment for fear the next moment would prove disappointing."

The following day, the two travelers rented a car and drove to Tahoe, where they planned to stay for two days, skiing and taking in the sights. Tammy, having been to Tahoe twice before, knew her way around and particularly knew the ski area where Mary Ellen would be most comfortable. At this point, Tammy said, "Mel was so excited as she realized she was finally here, in Tahoe. The months of anticipation had culminated and now the climax— Tahoe. However, she was coughing quite a bit, her stomach felt queasy, and she seemed rather tired. I begged her to call Dr. Guinan."

Mary Ellen refused because, as she reported later, "I was afraid the stomach pains were metastases."

Later on, when Dr. Guinan heard about the dilemma, she said, "I wish you had called. I could have assured you that the pains were certainly not metastases."

In any event they did get off to the slopes, but again Tammy noted that Mary Ellen, still coughing, seemed to become quite tired as they approached the lift. Tammy chose a moderate slope for the first run and as they started down, she noticed that Mary Ellen was not skiing well at all; in fact, she skied rather poorly. She had to stop a few times as they made their way down. Upon reaching the bottom, Tammy observed, "Mel was really pale and her breathing seemed labored. I suggested we sit in the sun for a while and relax. Just resting and observing all the fantastic sights—the people, the scenery, which was incredible—seemed to help as Mel started feeling a bit better. After a while, we went into the lodge for lunch and looked into the ski shop."

Tammy continued, "As we entered the ski shop, we suddenly heard a shout from one of the aisles. Around the corner came a young man who had seen us enter and who had also lost his leg

185

because of osteogenic sarcoma. Greg introduced himself to us, and he and Mary Ellen spent some time chatting and comparing notes about chemo as I skied. He was a great skier and was active with the Special Olympics Team. Mel also spent some time in the sun resting, and by late afternoon, she seemed to be feeling one hundred percent better."

After the Tahoe visit, the girls drove back to San Francisco to spend three days with Artie. Tammy said that Mary Ellen became more relaxed, stopped coughing, and truly seemed to be enjoying the sights.

Tammy, reflecting upon these two days, said she thought the excitement of the trip and any apprehensions Mary Ellen may have been experiencing probably caused the stomach pains. I think this was a pretty accurate assessment. Mary Ellen had looked forward to this trip for so long that she wanted nothing to interfere with it. She knew that the struggle was getting tougher and tougher and that she wasn't having much luck in winning the war. But she was in California now and she desperately tried to enjoy their vacation. As the days went by, she relaxed as she and Tammy spent the rest of their holiday seeing the sights of San Francisco.

They spent a day in Santa Cruz, lying on the beach and enjoying the beautiful scenery. They also took the 17-Mile Drive through the fantastic estates, viewing Pebble Beach and the Lone Cypress. The following day the girls toured San Francisco. As Tammy said, "Mel did great. We walked, rode the trolley cars, saw Fisherman's Wharf, took the boat trip to Alcatraz, and bought chocolate at Ghiradelli Square. She didn't seem to become tired, even though we walked and walked, She loved the trip to Alcatraz, which we investigated on our own, catching the last boat back to the Wharf." Tammy said Mary Ellen's thoughts on Alcatraz were: "This is great. I love it. How fantastic a place! This is something!"

As they approached the chocolate factory at the Square, it was the end of a perfect day and Mary Ellen was getting a bit tired. Walking up the steps, Tammy said all of a sudden Mary Ellen spotted a Benetton shop, her very favorite store. Up the stairs she went, heading right to the store, beating Tammy to the entrance. Tammy laughed and remarked, "If I had known what would have

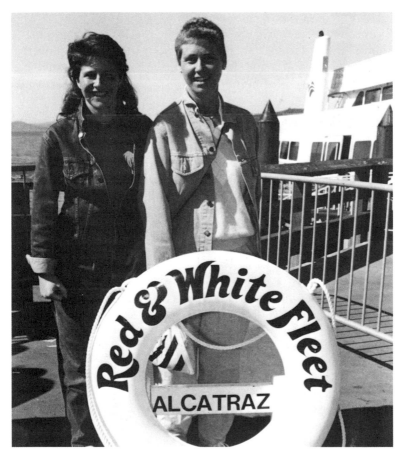

Tammy Jervas and Mary Ellen

made you really move, I would have waved a Benetton sign in front of you all the while."

Their last day in San Francisco was Mary Ellen's birthday, March 25. Artie showed them the city after dark, taking them on one of Artie's famous tours, reserved for all friends from the Berkshires. A lovely dinner at a restaurant situated on the water just about put the finishing touches to this most wonderful holiday. Tammy said Mary Ellen loved touring with Art. She thought it was absolutely the greatest and that Art was also the greatest.

Finally, about two in the morning, the three sightseers arrived back at Artie's, realizing the flight home would be in about eight hours. Tammy and Mary Ellen had sacked out when suddenly the lights came on and Artie, singing "Happy Birthday," carried in a cake he had baked for her. What a perfect end to a perfect vacation!

After Mary Ellen's death, Tammy and I spoke about the friendship that had existed between them. She said Mary Ellen did not discuss the "down" side of the disease with her, but rather, as Tammy noted, "She wanted me to be there for her; to be her friend. She didn't want to discuss treatments, but wanted to go out and have fun. Not that she avoided the subject, but that it was never brought up." Tammy then wrote to me and beautifully described her friendship with Mary Ellen:

I can't capture friendship on paper. Friendship is something untouchable and indescribable because it is not concrete. If I tried to describe Mel and our friendship, she would look perfect and angelic; neither of which any of us on this earth is.

Mel was my friend. We went to the same school, lived in the same county, did many of the same things. Unfortunately, when I went away for my first year at college, Mel went to the hospital for her first year of battle. She could not swing and hit; she could not run and hide; she had to stand tall and fight the "bugger" [as she called the cancer].

She knew she needed help, so she put her trust in her doctors and their knowledge and in her faith in a God she was raised to love. She believed in both of these with all her strength, and that's why she did so well against the bugger inside of her. There were ups and downs in Mel's battle, just like the ups and downs of our own lives. However, the ups were taken with a grain of salt and the downs were right hooks to the heart.

Mel was a big part of my life. She was a good friend. But I was dumb and did not realize how big she really was until I hugged her sister Katherine the day of Mel's funeral and she said to me, 'You were her best friend.' On the Friday before her death, when she lay there in the hospital bed in the den around 10:30 p.m., I was alone with Mel. I took her hand and said directly into her ear, 'Mel [her eyes opened], I love you very much and I am really going to miss you. I love you, Mel. I hope you know that.' I lifted my head from her ear and her eyes slowly shut as a tear ran down my face. I prayed she heard me. Even at that point, I hadn't realized who she was to me—my best friend.

What I want to say is simple and to the point. All of us should sit back away from work, away from everyday worries, and look at the people in our lives. Then picture what it would be like without them to go to the market, to share an ice cream cone, to share a laugh and a smile, a tear and a frown. Take no moment for granted, for we only pass by it once.

There's a lot more to our friendship. We shared a great deal—movies, laughs, plays, concerts, and more, much more, because all Mel really wanted was to be just like everyone else. To her, cancer was an inconvenience.

Whether she was Mary Ellen, Mel, or Mellon, she was certainly blessed with true friends—friends who cared and who shared with her every moment of her short life. She was blessed because her friends all played different roles, and when she needed to talk about a situation—be it a happy or sad one—there was a friend standing in the wings waiting for her, only too willing to listen or to share the moment. She did not have to struggle alone for one second of these five and a half years of battle, and for this we are grateful. We, her family, were her moral support, but her friends were her confidants.

> *Don't walk in front of me, I may not follow,*
> *Don't walk behind me, I may not lead,*
> *Just walk beside me and be my friend.*
> *Albert Camus*

4
❦

Upon returning from the "dream vacation," Mary Ellen went back to campus only to find herself becoming tired very easily. Dr. Guinan and the other doctors decided to try the Novobiocin protocol and Cyclophosphamide study to combat the existing tumors. it was explained to us that this was a Phase I study* with absolutely no guarantee of success and that an extremely limited number of patients had been treated. However, since Mary Ellen, as well as we, still felt the need for further treatment if there were a protocol available, we consented. Dr. Guinan again noted, "Mary Ellen is at her best during chemo since she thinks of it as a security blanket." She wasn't ready to give up just yet and still wanted to pursue any treatment that could perhaps slow down what was becoming increasingly clear as the inevitable. Each time she relapsed, Mary Ellen questioned Dr. Guinan, "What do you have in your bag of tricks now?"

Another plus for this treatment was that she had reacted well in the past to Cyclophosphamide drugs in the form of Ifosfamide. Reality, however, was setting in since it seemed as if nothing could stop the advancement of the disease. But again, as long as the drugs didn't seem to make her that nauseous and as long as she didn't have to miss weeks at a time from classes, Mary Ellen decided the treatments should take place.

Dr. Guinan wasn't just offering any treatment with the protocol, but rather a drug that had resulted in some success as the information in the introduction to Protocol 88-007 Cyclophosphamide and Novobiocin indicated:

> *Your cancer has recurred after standard chemotherapy or for which no standard chemotherapy exists. Further concentrational chemotherapy or radiation may be useful in this situation, but it is not likely to provide a long-term remission. This study uses a combination of a standard anti-cancer drug, Cyclophosphamide, along with an antibiotic, Novobiocin. Novobiocin has been used in the past to treat bacterial infections. Recent effectiveness has been noted of Cyclophosphamide against tumor cells without increasing the toxic effects of the drugs. The purpose of this study is to see if the Novobiocin can increase anti-tumor effects of chemotherapy drugs in patients without increasing the side effects of treatment.*

---

* A Phase I study means that rather than a set dosage, the amount of drug to be administered is determined by the toxicity occuring after the initial treatment. Therefore the dosage is altered depending upon the individual patient reaction.

After reading the protocol, we continued to hope that this drug might give Mary Ellen some more time with a remission. And again Dr. Guinan was constantly concerned with Mary Ellen's condition as she continuously strived to search out chemo protocols that could possibly help. We knew that all the knowledge to fight the disease was there at the Dana-Farber or within reach of it, so we left the continuing battle to their expertise. If there were a possible solution to the disease, the medical staff would be there for us.

With this protocol, Mary Ellen had to take the antibiotic Novobiocin every twelve hours for two days before the start of the chemotherapy. Early one morning in April, I met a friend, Ann Makuc, at the turnpike and we drove to Boston so I could pick up the Novobiocin. We arrived at 8:30, received the prescription from Dr. Guinan, had it filled at the pharmacy, and started back. We reached the college before noon, so Mary Ellen could begin taking the medication. She would continue with the antibiotic for the two days, and then the chemo. Besides taking the antibiotic, Mary Ellen had to give two quarts of "pee" before she could be approved. The urine was tested at Baystate and the results, which were only just favorable, sent to Boston. With all of these preliminaries out of the way, we hoped she would have an effective treatment. Mary Ellen remained at the college, trying to keep up with her classes while going through these initial procedures.

When we discussed the administering of the chemo, Dr. Guinan had at first stated that with a new Children's Hospital, all the chemo patients were to be treated on the same floor so Mary Ellen probably could not go to her old friends of Division 36, now 10 North. There was also the possibility she'd have to be treated at the Dana-Farber. This news didn't sit very well with her as she said, "I really want to have the nurses on 36 give me the chemo."

When we arrived at the Clinic the day of the treatment, Dr. Guinan said, "Report to 10 North!" Mary Ellen was so happy to be with her old friends and to see their new quarters, now that the old had moved into the new. Once again Dr. Guinan "pulled a few strings," thinking only of Mary Ellen's welfare. Since she had to be in the hospital for the chemo, she didn't mind if she could be with the nurses who meant so much to her. Hospitalization was necessary in case of vomiting in which case oral medication could not be given and an IV would prove necessary. Since Mary Ellen weathered the chemo well, not becoming nauseous, she was discharged the following day.

5
❦

JIMMY AND I STAYED AT MARGARET'S WHILE MARY ELLEN underwent the chemo. Dr. Guinan had arranged for the treatment over the weekend so she wouldn't miss any activities at school. Since everything proceeded well, we left Boston April 18 to return to Sheffield. Mary Ellen planned to spend the day home resting and to return to campus the following morning. The upcoming weekend at Springfield was the big Sty-U-Ka Spring Fling, beginning with a concert on Thursday. Mary Ellen had been looking forward to all of the activities and was most anxious to be a part of the weekend. Since this week was Mount Everett's spring vacation, Jimmy and I had planned to visit Katherine at MWC and our cousins, the Barringers, near Washington, D.C., perhaps playing golf in Fredericksburg.

We were a bit nervous about leaving now for Virginia, since Mary Ellen obviously was not feeling the greatest, but we knew that canceling our trip would indeed bother her. Again, the knowledge that she would be well taken care of at the college; that Jim Jr. would be at home, a phone call away; and that Kelly and Joe Milan had offered assistance if the need arose, convinced us to keep our plans intact.

On April 19, early in the morning, we drove Mary Ellen to Springfield and then started on our way to Virginia. She was excited about the spring weekend as she happily returned to the dorm and told us goodbye: "Have a great time. Say hi to Kack [our nickname for Katherine] and the Barringers. Call me when you get home on Sunday." We wished her a great weekend as we left the campus, hoping it would prove to be a fun one for her.

We enjoyed a game of golf on the Fredericksburg course and did some sightseeing in D.C. and Georgetown with Katherine. She showed us the restaurant where she and Jen hoped to work during the summer, since they had definitely decided to spend the summer in Georgetown. She also pointed out the condo they would share with two other girls from MWC. We had lunch in a Georgetown landmark, the Toombs, and even saw the University basketball coach, John Thompson, enjoying his lunch a few tables from ours. On Friday, April 22, when we returned to Katherine's room after having done some shopping, Jen called to say Mary Ellen had called from Springfield to tell us she was okay but rather tired and would be going to Kelly's that afternoon. Andy and Wendy would drive her, and we weren't to worry.

Not to worry? How could we not be concerned? I immediately called Kelly, who assured us that Mary Ellen was all right, but felt that the activities during the remainder of the week would be too tiring. I talked with her, "I didn't want to be a drag for the kids the rest of the weekend, so I thought I'd come to Kelly's." She kept repeating, "I'm okay. Don't cut your vacation short." Rather than make her feel bad by coming home earlier than planned, we compromised. "We'll stay another day here and then come home Saturday. The Barringers will understand if we cut out that part of our trip."

Kelly later told me about Mary Ellen's decision to return home rather than stay for the rest of the weekend.

She called me Thursday and said, 'I don't feel well. I'm tired. I'm having trouble breathing. I feel awful,' I told her I'd come get her but she retorted, 'No, there's the concert tonight. I have my ticket and I really want to go.'

We decided that if during the night she began to feel much worse, she'd call me, and my sister, Nora, and I would drive to Springfield. She did call the next day to tell us that Wendy and Andy would drive her to our house.

She was in good spirits but said, 'I don't feel good.' She lay on the couch and really didn't feel like going anywhere or doing anything. Every time I'd ask her, she'd say, 'I'm too tired.'

That evening as we ate dinner, you guys called and she kept saying, 'Tell my father I'm eating. He worries that I'm not eating.' She did eat her dinner and then Jim Jr. went home, but she decided to stay the night with us.

The next morning I tried to keep Corey from bothering her, but he finally crawled in bed with her and they lay there talking. She and Corey watched cartoons and sort of hung out together the rest of the day, when Jim Jr. came to take her home since you guys were expected later in the afternoon.

After Mary Ellen's death, Kelly remarked to me, "I had wondered what part I was to play in Mary Ellen's struggle. Where did I fit into the scheme of things. As the disease was taking its toll, I

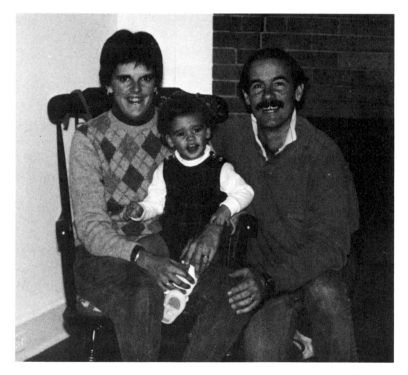

Kelly, Corey and Joe

194

realized what my role was. Mary Ellen could come to our house and flop on the couch and be herself. She didn't have to smile, but could be content just to hang out and not feel she had to do things and go places. Our house was sort of an island of rest and repose, away from the excitement of campus and away from the worried looks of you and Jimmy."

When we arrived home later in the day, Mary Ellen was there, tired and content to just lie on the couch. She said, "The concert was great, but with all the partying going on, I'd be too tired to be much fun." She seemed glad to be home as we assured her our trip had been fun and we really didn't mind coming home a day early.

"The extra day will give me a chance to catch up on my homework," I kidded. We didn't talk much about her returning to campus on Monday when she was also due for the usual blood test that followed chemo. We decided to wait to see how she felt before deciding whether she'd return to classes.

On Monday we went to Springfield for the blood test. Mary Ellen decided to return to campus and try to go to classes and to attend the Awards Night program because Amy and Julie would be receiving many of the awards. Amy remembered this evening as she said, "There 'Jools' [Julie] and I were with all of these awards as Mary Ellen came up and just hugged me. She started crying hysterically and I too cried. I questioned her, 'Mary Ellen, what is it?' 'Oh, Aim, I'm never going to see this again. I'm never going to see this again,' Mary Ellen sobbed."

Amy described the moment, "Her cane dropped. She just collapsed."

Mary Ellen continued to sob, "Aim, I saw you through every single one of these awards."

"Mellon," Amy cried, "I know, I know. I owe most of it to you." Amy continued, "Her tears wouldn't stop and I just wanted to hold her up. She had become thinner and frailer."

The day after the Awards Night, Mary Ellen called to say things weren't going well, and she felt she should come home. She was finding it increasingly difficult to attend classes, as she experienced a throbbing pain in the upper left shoulder and back area, preventing her from sleeping. I went to campus to get her. While on campus, I checked with the registrar's office about her taking incompletes in her courses. They said this could be done, and if she felt better during the summer, she could contact the professors to complete the courses. With this taken care of, she seemed a bit happier, knowing she wouldn't get F's. We didn't talk about packing all of her things and leaving the campus for good, but rather we just treated this like a minor setback and that she'd return sometime soon. She was especially disappointed that she was feeling so tired since Colleen Hax had invited her to attend a Michael Jackson concert in Connecticut the following week. Mary Ellen, however, took the disappointment in her stride. As we drove home, she did mention her back and said, "Now if I had a water bed, I probably could sleep a bit better." She had talked about getting a water bed, but we never gave her any encouragement, probably because the floor in her bedroom couldn't handle the weight.

6
❧

THE NEXT APPOINTMENT WITH DR. GUINAN WAS APRIL 29, 1988. Dr. Guinan's notes for that date give a clear picture of Mary Ellen's condition, as we watched her become progressively thinner and more tired. Her prosthesis began giving her problems because of the weight loss and, as only Mary Ellen could put it, "Losing weight makes my leg fart as I walk. Sometimes it's embarrassing!"

Dr. Guinan's notes for the April 29 visit:

Mary Ellen tolerated the chemo extremely well and the blood tests have been good. She will return Friday, May 6, for a repeat chest X-ray and to assess the progress of therapy. In addition, I have spoken to both Mary Ellen and her parents separately on the telephone on multiple occasions in this interval, particularly in the last two weeks. As regards the patient, she is depressed, but is verbalizing her concerns and is certainly realistic in terms of knowing that her time is quite limited. She does address this directly. A typical comment would be that she knows that she will not be around for Spring Weekend next year unless something quite extraordinary happens. Her major complaint at this point is a sore and somewhat throbbing back in the region of her previous surgery when she goes to sleep at night. We have attempted to treat this with Advil without significant relief and she is at present discussing this with Dr. Kelleher. My impression would be that she'd benefit from some Valium and Advil, although she may perhaps need a more powerful analgesia. As to her parents, I have discussed with them, particularly Mrs. Welch, in great detail, the fact that there is still some potential, as there was in the past, that something catastrophic could happen. Her tumor could either forcefully invade her spinal canal, erode into a blood vessel or other major structure, or she could have some major catastrophic clotting event. We have gone over this in order to prepare the family for this eventuality, although I have stressed that I think that it is reasonably unlikely. Mrs. Welch states that she understands that this is a possibility and also understands that there is very little that we can do to guard against it.

The prognosis now ominously put forth the thought that an extraordinary event needs to occur if Mary Ellen is to continue to enjoy life. So it had finally come down to the fact that a miraculous occurrence must take place or Mary Ellen will die. As I spoke with Dr. Guinan at the end of April, and as she told me what I really knew deep down in my heart and soul, we could only pray that the worst would not occur, and if death were to come, it would do so without agony and pain, but rather quietly and with comfort and dignity. Mary Ellen had, from what Wendy indicated, come to the realization that her time was definitely limited. She had resolved all issues and I believe had taken solace and comfort in knowing that we would remain at her side for as long as she needed us. She would not, however, discuss the final stage with us since, I'm certain, she had come to an acceptance of her approaching death and wanted to spare us, her family, further grief and anxiety. This was her way and we accepted it. The only reference she made to her dying occurred as Dr. Guinan questioned her, "Do you want to be at home or in the hospital the last days?"

197

Mary Ellen quietly answered, "I want to be at home with my family and friends." This seemed to close the door on any further discussion.

7
❦

KATHERINE FINISHED THE SEMESTER THE END OF APRIL AND returned home with all of her paraphernalia. She unpacked and sorted out clothes in preparation for the trip with Jen to Georgetown. One morning she asked, "Do you think I should stay home this summer?"

I could only answer, "No one knows for certain what will happen, and you'll be just an hour away by plane if we need you. I can't tell you to stay home, nor can I tell you to go." I felt that I couldn't, in all honesty, plan Katherine's summer for her.

Not satisfied with my response, Katherine talked to her second mother, Sue Kinsley, Jen's mom. She could be more direct and so insisted, "You stay home. Don't go to Georgetown."

Katherine and Jen decided to follow her advice. Later in the day, Katherine told me, "Jen and I will stay home and be with Mary Ellen this summer. We'll take her places and do things." I was secretly very happy with their decision.

When she told Mary Ellen of her change in plans, Mary Ellen came to me and asked, "Does she know something I don't?"

I assured Mary Ellen we all knew exactly what she knew; no more, no less. This was indeed true since Dr. Guinan was very frank and open with Mary Ellen and with us. Katherine's decision to remain at home was obviously on her mind when she spoke with Wendy as the two of them got ready to leave campus for the summer. Wendy indicated to me that the room was bare, they were packed to go, and Mary Ellen told her, "Katherine has changed her plans and will be home for the summer. I think she knows something I don't know."

Mary Ellen, however, was so happy that Katherine chose to remain at home, and she revealed this thought to Tammy Jervas. During the last weeks of Mary Ellen's life, she and Katherine spent the time together, becoming even closer in their relationship. Katherine, too, felt the bond deepening between them as they were together as much as possible. Katherine indeed proved to be a sister in the true sense of the word.

8

ON FRIDAY, MAY 6, WE RETURNED TO THE CLINIC FOR THE follow-up after the last chemo. The chest X-ray indicated some regrowth of tumor, so obviously the Novobiocin protocol had been to no avail. As Dr. Guinan checked the lump on Mary Ellen's arm, which had gotten progressively larger and more pronounced, she decided the radiation people should also take a look. One of Dr. Tarbell's assistants, Dr. Bornstein, consulted with Dr. Guinan, and they decided a series of radiation treatments would be in order to try to attack the growth of the lump, which they now decided was a metastatic lesion. The radiation would begin on May 16. As we left Dr. Guinan's office, Mary Ellen again asked her, "What do you have in your bag of tricks now?"

Dr. Guinan answered, "After we take care of the radiation, we'll talk about what's next." Dr. Guinan gave me a knowing glance and put her arm around my shoulder as we left her office. Our good friends in Clinic—Mary, Susan, Irene—and all of the others knew from our faces that things weren't progressing too well. We said our goodbyes and left to go to 10 North to visit the nurses. In a week's time we would return to the Brigham to begin the radiation process again.

I'm certain that some readers might wonder, "Why all of the

chemo and radiation when the treatments obviously did not stop the growth of the cancer? Why did Mary Ellen subject herself to these different protocols?" She was not ready to give up yet. She had to keep fighting: mentally, physically, and emotionally. She knew her time on this earth was limited, but she could not just sit back and not fight as long as Dr. Guinan and the others at the Jimmy Fund Clinc could recommend a drug that might possibly stop the growth. There were protocols that Dr. Guinan would not give her stamp of approval to simply because they were too radical. If there were a protocol, however, that might give her more quality time and that would not cause her to be so sick she would be confined to bed, Mary Ellen wanted to know about it. We knew that when the time came that there would be no more treatments, we would all be prepared to accept the inevitable. But until that point in our battle, we would continue to fight.

During the following week, we visited Dr. Kelleher for medication to try to ease the discomfort in Mary Ellen's back. The Springfield campus was in the midst of exams and since Mary Ellen certainly wasn't ready for them, she decided to pack up her things. One afternoon we drove to the campus and collected everything. She had decided in March, when room assignments for the fall were being processed, to live in a house off campus with Carolyn Grant and two or three other girls. We did not waver in these plans, again sincerely hoping for that miraculous occurrence. Wendy, still undecided about her living arrangements since she would be doing a great deal of fieldwork, thought she would probably find an apartment off campus. We all knew that Mary Ellen might not be back in September, but such thoughts were never uttered as we went about the task of packing. We left with promises of seeing the girls at graduation on May 22 and of visiting during the summer.

9

AS THE WEEK CAME TO A CLOSE, MARY ELLEN PLANNED TO GO with us to a retirement party for one of our good friends and a fellow teacher, Leo Alvares. She started to rise from the chair to get ready for the party, using her crutches. As she leaned on them, an excruciating pain shot up her arm and she screamed in anguish. The lesion or lump in her arm had evidently resulted in nerve compression, causing the pain. She sobbed as Jimmy and I both went running to her. I quickly called the page number at Children's and in two minutes spoke with Dr. Guinan, who said, "I'll call you back very shortly. Be prepared to leave for Boston and we'll try for emergency radiation to begin Saturday morning at the Brigham. Give Mary Ellen some Motrin or Advil for the pain."

We quickly packed a few things, made a few phone calls, told Jimmy and Katherine the plan, and awaited Dr. Guinan's call. In a very short time she phoned. "All is set for radiation at the Brigham tomorrow morning at 9. They will do the emergency treatment Saturday and Sunday, and on Monday will do the plotting and charting for the rest of the sessions, again probably three weeks in duration."

We thanked her and were on our way to Margaret's in Boston that evening, in preparation for the treatment early the next day.

The Advil helped and the pain subsided. As we drove along the turnpike, we thought, "What next?" It just seemed as if our whole world was crumbling before our very eyes. Mary Ellen always became angry with herself if she showed any sign of giving in to crying or moaning, but she certainly had every right to do so as we traveled toward what would be another session of treatments. I'm sure the thoughts of amputation of her arm if the radiation didn't work were uppermost in her mind. I know they were in mine. But as we had done in the past, we decided to try to think positively, commenting on the good results she had experienced with previous radiation treatments. And again we marveled at the quick response from Dr. Guinan, who had never failed us. We arrived at the Brigham about 9 o'clock Saturday morning. Since radiation treatments weren't usually done on Saturdays, it was very quiet as we awaited Dr. Hiaasen and the technician.

Since Mary Ellen had lost some weight, Oliver did not fit too well and she had to resort to using the crutches, which put a decided strain on her arm. However, after the treatment on Sunday, her arm began to feel a bit better. Jimmy and I decided we would not share the days in Boston, but rather I would stay with Mary Ellen since she had difficulty getting dressed. On Monday, after the charting (the procedure to determine the exact area to be radiated), Mary Ellen, Jimmy, and I were able to return home for a day so I could get my classes in order for my substitute, Peggy Muskrat. John Peron, the head of the language department at Mount Everett, and Peggy were more than helpful in taking over for me so I had no worries about my classes. My students were very cooperative and could be counted on to do their all in this latest emergency.

Each morning Mary Ellen and I reported to the Brigham at 7 o'clock for radiation and then went back to the apartment until 2 o'clock, when we returned for the second daily treatment. After the morning session, Mary Ellen usually took a nap as I read the paper and caught up with paperwork. At 9 o'clock I made my daily call to Mount Everett. At this time I spoke with Peggy or whoever else was subbing for me, and then I chatted with any of my students who might be having problems with the assignments. As I checked in with my students and the office, Mary Ellen would laugh as she commented, "I don't believe you are conducting classes over the phone! What next!"

During this week, we spent time sitting in the park, watching the kids fly kites, shopping and visiting. Dan Andrus and Betsy Aloisi, two of Mary Ellen's friends, were to be married the end of June so one afternoon after a treatment, Mary Ellen suggested, "Let's go to Cherry, Webb, and Touraine in Brookline so I can buy a dress and shoes for the wedding. I need a new bathing suit, too." We had a leisurely lunch and then went to the shop. We searched out a suitable dress before trying any on since Mary Ellen tired easily now, and trying on a lot of clothes wasn't too much fun. As we bought the outfit, I couldn't help but think that Mary Ellen's going to this wedding probably wouldn't be possible. Again I said nothing, since I knew how much she was looking forward to the wedding and seeing all of her old skiing buddies. Perhaps she struggled with the same thoughts as I did now, but with her determination, as in the past, maybe she would get to go.

From the very beginning of our struggle, we never stopped planning, nor did we ever give in to "What if?" or "Maybe you'd better not." We made plans and always looked ahead. If we had to cancel an event, we did so with an alternative date always in mind. Again, it was rare that we ever canceled since Mary Ellen had such intense determination.

During the week, Mary Ellen spoke with Wendy, Amy, and the others at Springfield. Amy, Julie, and Andy were to graduate on Sunday, May 22, and Mary Ellen told them we'd be there. As the week drew to a close, we noted that the lump was decreasing in size and the pressure on her arm was diminishing. The radiation treatments were having the effect we all hoped for. After the treatment on Friday afternoon, we drove home for the weekend, to return on Sunday after Amy's graduation.

We relaxed Saturday and planned to attend the graduation at 11 Sunday morning in the Springfield Civic Center. Mary Ellen had been sleeping in our bedroom downstairs, since we thought this arrangement would be best for her. She found herself being more and more tired, and getting out of bed took longer now. We did not rush Sunday to make the graduation, but decided just to go to Amy's party held at Ken Childs' home near the college. Amy's family was all there, as well as some faculty members. We enjoyed the festivities and then made our return trip to Margaret's, since radiation treatments would continue during the week. Mary Ellen was able to wear Oliver, even though he did not fit so well. She usually felt better wearing her leg. That Sunday afternoon she was in good spirits as she renewed her acquaintance with Amy's family.

10

🍂

DURING THE NEXT WEEK, WE FOLLOWED THE SAME ROUTINE. We did go to dinner at Aunt Frances' one evening, finding our way to Arlington with Mary Ellen reading the map to me. The lesion was definitely getting smaller, and we were thankful for the radiation easing the pain while taking care of the growth of the tumor. However, the notes from the Brigham on May 25 revealed Mary Ellen's condition as extremely serious:

> *Thoracic back pain, stiffness, lower rib pain particularly early morning. Taking Dilaudid and Advil. Mary Ellen becomes easily fatigued. She has been pushing herself to get through treatments and often lies down at home in between treatments. She is planning on attending a friend's wedding this weekend and visiting with family.*

At the end of the week, May 27, we met with Dr. Guinan after the morning radiation treatment. The notes from this appointment also indicates the seriousness of Mary Ellen's condition:

> *Mary Ellen continues to have difficulty. Her left antecubital lesion has been radiated with relatively good result. She has full strength in that hand. She has no numbness or tingling. She is able to use her crutches and to ambulate without difficulty. She continues to have modest weight loss and continues to have pain in her left lung, site of tumor. She also has some symptoms; i.e. right shoulder pain, referable to diaphragmatic mass on that side. Although chest X-ray today shows no significant change, we can only assume that her tumor is continuing to grow. She will complete her radiation next week and will return to see me one week thereafter. I again discussed with her parents issues surrounding the fact that the patient is, in fact, dying and that there is certainly some risk for her to have an acute hemorrhagic or thrombotic event.*

Jimmy and I worried about the possibly of the hemorrhaging to which Dr. Guinan referred in her notes. Being informed helped, since we now prepared ourselves for this possible development.

We sincerely hoped and prayed, however, that this terrible ordeal would not occur and that God in His infinite mercy would protect Mary Ellen from so disastrous an end. We prayed that when death came, it would do so peacefully and without pain.

11
❧

FRIDAY, MAY 27, CONCLUDED ANOTHER WEEK OF RADIATION. We planned to return home after the 2 o'clock treatment, but before the treatment Mary Ellen said, "I really feel like Chinese food. Let's go to China Sails [a restaurant in Chestnut Hill]."

Her appetite was not so great, so I hesitated and answered, "Why don't we just stay here at Margaret's and have tuna fish?"

"I'll eat, really," she promised.

So despite the rain, we decided to try the restaurant. As we approached it, we could find no place to park within easy walking distance. Going around the block for the second time, Mary Ellen said, "Park there." She pointed to a bank parking area with the sign "For customers only. Violators will be towed." When I pointed out the sign, Mary Ellen laughed, "There's no one parked there. Go ahead." We left the car and walked quickly to the restaurant.

We ordered, but when our lunch came, Mary Ellen ate a few bites and said, "I guess I'm not really very hungry." She ate a little more and then we told the waiter we'd take the rest home for dinner. After paying the bill, I left Mary Ellen waiting in front of the restaurant as I ran up the street to get the car. In the parking lot there were two cars, neither of them ours. "Oh, my God," I moaned as I ran into the bank, completely empty of customers, and spoke to one of the tellers. "I parked my car in the lot about thirty minutes ago and it's not there now. Please help me!"

She took a minute from her conversation with the other teller and answered matter-of-factly, "It probably got towed."

"Towed," I yelled. "Why?"

She explained, "The lot is for our customers only."

By now I was panicky as I exclaimed, "I have a daughter who is due for a radiation treatment in about thirty minutes at the Brigham Hospital. She is not feeling well and how do you suppose I'm to get her to the hospital? Besides, there was a handicap plate on the car. Not that that should give us any privileges, but why didn't they just give us a ticket?"

I guess my performance was worthy of an Academy Award because the tellers got together and called the towing company. I spoke to the person in charge, telling him my tale of woe. He called the tow truck (thank God for car phones), telling the driver to return the car to the bank parking lot.

When I asked the cost, the dispatcher said, "Forty dollars."

I exclaimed at the price, so he countered with "Twenty-five dollars."

In the meantime, poor Mary Ellen waited at the restaurant. I ran back, filled her in on all the details, and since she felt nauseous, we quickly walked to the bank.

"May my daughter use your rest room? She's not feeling too well," I questioned the tellers.

Mary Ellen now had to walk down two flights of stairs to the bathroom. I settled her there and then ran back upstairs to await the tow truck and the car. Finally the car arrived and I paid the driver, who really wasn't too happy about the whole situation. The only thing I said to him was, "Where we come from, nobody tows cars." I went down to the bathroom and helped Mary Ellen up the stairs. We left the parking lot and headed for the hospital and friendlier territory, where the parking is made easier by very courteous attendants.

When we told our tale to Verona Brooks and the others at Radiation, they didn't know whether to laugh or cry. By this time, we were laughing about our mishap as we said to each other, "Wait till Daddy finds out!" After the treatment, we started on our way home. Since Monday was Memorial Day, there would be no treatment until Tuesday, May 31. Again as we drove home, Mary Ellen reminded me, "Never a dull moment when you're with me!"

12

ON SATURDAY MORNING MARY ELLEN'S HIGH SCHOOL CLASS-
mate Laurie Briggs was to be married. Mary Ellen and I had
planned to attend, but when the morning arrived and Mary Ellen
felt too tired to get dressed for the wedding, I went as planned. It
was getting more and more difficult for her to get going in the
morning. She had to take her time to get ready since putting on
Oliver became more difficult because her strength was waning and
the weight loss made a good fit impossible. Laurie and her family
had followed Mary Ellen's progress these many years and knew that
if she could have come, she would have. When I returned in the
early afternoon, Mary Ellen and Danielle had gone out to lunch. She
had gotten her second wind, so to speak. Mary Ellen rarely passed
up an opportunity to go to lunch or shopping, especially with
Danielle, who with her husband was now stationed in Norfolk.

The following day, Sunday, I spoke with our pastor, Father
Heberle, after Mass. He mentioned that he'd like to stop by to visit
with Mary Ellen later in the morning. I said, "That would be great.
I'm sure she would like to see you."

He always remembered Mary Ellen in the prayers during Mass.
We appreciated his thoughtfulness, but as Mary Ellen indicated, "It
could and did prove embarrassing, especially when Father prayed
for me and there I was!" Many times during the years of struggle she
would be in the hospital and then return before anyone realized.
Sometimes we didn't get a chance to tell Father she was back home
or in school, so he'd pray for her, not realizing immediately that
Mary Ellen was in the congregation.

Later, when I mentioned her feelings about the prayers, Father
said, "I'll look around before I begin Mass to be sure she's not
present." Father was always considerate and caring, and constantly
asked about Mary Ellen's health.

13

🍂

ON MEMORIAL DAY WE PLANNED TO GO TO HILLSDALE, WHERE my brother Donald's nursery was having a picnic, and then to Kelly and Joe's for hamburgers. The following day Mary Ellen and I were to return to Boston to begin the last week of radiation treatments. Mary Ellen decided that morning that she really did not feel like the trip back to Boston for the last four days of treatment, especially since her arm was just about back to normal and there was no longer any pain. I called Dr. Guinan and then Dr. Tarbell to tell them of Mary Ellen's decision. Since we were to see Dr. Guinan on Friday, June 3, Dr. Tarbell suggested that we also report to Radiation, where she could administer a final treatment. Both Dr. Guinan and Dr. Tarbell respected Mary Ellen's decision, and I believe they agreed with her. I think at this point Mary Ellen came to the conclusion that there would be no more treatments. She had accepted the fact that unless an extraordinary event occurred, her days were definitely limited. She was just too tired to cope any more with all that the treatments would entail.

The weather cooperated this Memorial Day, as we went first to Kelly's and visited for a while, enjoying lunch. Later that afternoon found us at Hillsdale, where the nursery employees engaged in their yearly volleyball tournament: garden shop versus landscapers. Jim Jr. was already there doing battle for the garden center champs. Mary Ellen sat in Grandpa's chair on the patio and surveyed the festivities. She turned to me and said, "It's so great here. Let's plan to spend the summer here at Grandpa's." We all experienced an emptiness in Hillsdale, since this was the first Memorial Day without Nanny and Grandpa, but the memories we shared were happy ones. Jimmy and I agreed to spend the summer and Mary Ellen also suggested, "Let's invite Aunt Rita and Aunt Marian. They always loved spending the summer here with Nanny and Grandpa." And so, our plans for the summer made, we looked forward to the peace and quiet of Hillsdale.

14

❧

DURING THE WEEK, MARY ELLEN AND KATHERINE ENJOYED the laziness of no school and no books. On June 1, Mary Ellen went to Sharon Hospital for a routine chest X-ray as we planned to go to Boston June 3 for an appointment with Dr. Guinan. Katherine decided to go to Boston with us and since Oliver was not really fitting too well and to make the day easier for Mary Ellen, we took the wheelchair that my mother had used. Our first appointment was at the Jimmy Fund Clinic. Katherine had great fun pushing the wheelchair with complete abandon, so we arrived breathless from laughing. Dr. Guinan's notes from this visit are quite explicit regarding Mary Ellen's condition at this time:

Mary Ellen comes in acutely worse. Over the past four or five days she has had some modestly increased shortness of breath. Chest X-ray was performed per my recommendation, which showed no evidence of any acute event; i.e. pneumothorax. She had not had a fever, although she is producing somewhat more sputum, and of note her white count is somewhat elevated today at 17.7. I therefore think it would be worthwhile to give her a course of Erythromycin. Otherwise, she was given an extra large dose of radiation to her left arm, and I don't feel it is necessary that she have further radiation to this extremity unless the lesion again begins growing. Issues around her pain care, a bowel regimen, etc. were discussed with the parents and the patient in detail. I will discuss her with Dr. Gallup and she will come back on a schedule which depends on the future course of events.

The future course of events remained a mystery to us. We knew as we left the Clinic that there was nothing left for Dr. Guinan to prescribe in the way of treatment, and we knew that ultimately we were going to lose Mary Ellen, but we also had no idea of what was to come, either immediately or later on. As we left, Mary Ellen, wanting to keep the moment as light as possible, said to Dr. Guinan, "What's left in the bag of tricks?" No one could answer her question. I'm certain Mary Ellen knew the answer, but again wanted to keep the mood from being a depressing one.

With Katherine pushing the wheelchair, still in a carefree fashion, we headed down the street to the Brigham and the final dose of radiation. Verona Brooks, an assistant in the radiation department, and Dr. Tarbell's nurse, Kathy, were a bit surprised to see the change in Mary Ellen since the preceding week. Dr. Tarbell administered the dose and we said our farewells, leaving to go to lunch and then home. This would be our last appointment with the Boston people, a fact that we did not know at that time. Thank God we didn't. We could not have experienced the day of goodbyes that this knowledge would have precipitated. Instead we left, very upbeat and laughing, without any mournful farewells. This is the way Mary Ellen was. She wanted no one to cry for her, but rather to remember her smiling and enjoying life to its fullest.

Upon our return home, Mary Ellen seemed to experience more and more difficulty in breathing. We had discussed this with the doctors, and it was decided that some oxygen would help. I called an organization in Great Barrington that helps with terminal patients. Barbara Dolby, the nurse in charge, was a great help as she gave me phone numbers to call so we could get the portable oxygen tanks. I called Wayne Speyrer, a nurse associated with Barbara, who came to our assistance. We got the oxygen, and with a lesson from Wayne regarding its use, Mary Ellen felt a bit more comfortable since breathing wasn't so difficult now. Since the tank was portable, Mary Ellen could go out in the car and attend some of the graduation functions. The pain in her back was more and more evident as we tried all sorts of remedies. Nothing seemed to help, but we did decide to have the hospital bed that my mother had used brought from Hillsdale and set up in the TV room, hoping to make Mary Ellen more comfortable, especially at night.

15

🍂

THE MOUNT EVERETT GRADUATION TOOK PLACE ON SATURDAY, June 2, at Tanglewood in Lenox. We were invited to many parties but declined since Mary Ellen was content to rest and relax at home. On June 3, Colleen Ward, our niece, graduated from Monument Mountain High School in Great Barrington. We did go to Colleen's party later in the afternoon. Mary Ellen now used the oxygen continuously, as well as the wheelchair, since the weight loss affected Oliver's normally good fit. She was in a down mood as we arrived at the Wards', but soon her spirts picked up and she chatted with her cousins and friends. A little boy, whose father, Gordon Clark, works at Ward's Nursery, seemed intrigued with Mary Ellen's lack of a leg, since he, too, had a small prosthesis from the knee down. Mary Ellen spoke to him, "I have one of those, too," she said, pointing to his prosthesis.

A friend, Jean Tomich, wrote after Mary Ellen's death, remembering this day:

> Just a short note to let you all know that you are often in our thoughts and prayers. I pray that God is sustaining you with the same strength that you displayed during those so sorrowful days. I'm sure the emptiness and sadness you feel must be almost unbearable at times.
>
> Your child was very special and taught us what courage means, especially that day of Colleen's party. That's something none of us will forget and the memory of the way she faced death will hopefully help us when our time comes.

Coleen Cecchinato, a student at Mount Everett who first met Mary Ellen one summer while on a bus trip to Yankee Stadium (Mary Ellen, Jimmy, and Jim Jr. took advantage of a tour sponsored by the Knights of Columbus, as did Coleen and her father), wrote an English assignment the September after Mary Ellen died:

The picture I am most intrigued by is the picture of my friend Miss Mary Ellen Welch that hangs above my bed. This picture was taken before Mary Ellen had become so very ill. It reminds me of how brave she was. When I'm sad or depressed, I always look at the picture of her because it says to me that nothing I ever go through will be as hard or as upsetting as that which this young woman went through.

Mary Ellen's confidant and roommate at Springfield, Amy Kissel, while a senior at the college, wrote an essay entitled, "A Woman Making History—My Role Model," depicting the strength Mary Ellen demonstrated during the good times and the bad times:

She is the world's toughest competitor. In her five years of formal competition, she has never received a medal, trophy, honorable mention, certificate, or M.V.P. award for her achievements. In her own right, however, she is a champion and deserves to be on the Wheaties boxes of the world.

Who is this outstanding competitor? She is a friendly, outgoing woman who rarely complains about all of the pain, sweat, and suffering her training puts her through. The passion she feels for competition is evident in her unwillingness to quit. To completely understand the drives of this woman, one must examine her daily fitness regimen and her underlying philosophy of life.

She goes into each of her competitions with the most optimistic attitude possible. She has lost and she has sacrificed, but her intense competitive drive had not been altered. 'Who knows?' she once said. 'I may not be here for tomorrow's performance, so I'll do the best that I possibly can today.' By facing the workout or the competition at hand, without looking back or worrying about future events, she allowed herself the opportunity to turn each moment into a performance of a lifetime and she succeeds. She is a true champion.

...Presently this woman is a Junior Rehabilitation Major at Springfield College. She plans on using her competitive experience in the future, as a rehabilitation counselor at Boston Children's Hospital, her home away from home. Interestingly, Mary Ellen has turned this biological disaster into something worthwhile to humanity. She believes she was given the gift of cancer for a reason. 'Sure, I've questioned why and I've felt sorry for myself, but then I realized that crying didn't change the potential positive impact that I can have on the world.' She is a woman living for now and for improvements in the future; she is a woman making history.

212

Perhaps Mary Ellen will not make it onto the Wheaties box, but there is no doubt that she will make it in this world as she accepts the challenges each day brings her way.

It was now obvious that Mary Ellen would not "make it in this world," but we had the consolation that her presence in this world, even for a brief twenty-two years, had a profound effect on many persons, several we know, but so many we'll not know in this lifetime.

After the weekend, I returned to my students at Mount Everett to find that Peggy and John had indeed carried on for me in my absence. However, my students were concerned about their final exams, so we spent Monday and Tuesday reviewing and outlining exam material. Mary Ellen seemed to be doing well with the portable oxygen, and Katherine provided the entertainment as they went out in the car or just sat around watching the "soaps." Tuesday evening, June 7, Mary Ellen, rather dejected that she hadn't been out of the house that day, said, "I've got to get out. Let's go for a ride." Jimmy, Katherine, Mary Ellen, and I drove through the back roads of Sheffield, Mill River, and Hartsville, arriving at the Friendly's in Great Barrington, where we all had extra large ice cream cones. When we reached home, we rubbed Mary Ellen's back with Ben-Gay to ease the discomfort she felt because of the tumor in the upper left lung. Dr. Kelleher had prescribed some pain medication, which she took before going to sleep.

16

❧

THE NEXT DAY DR. GUINAN CONTACTED DR. GALLUP, ASKING him to check in on Mary Ellen, which he did, spending a few hours with her, talking and listening as she confided to him her anxieties and fears of what was to come. Later that morning, Dr. Gallup called me at school, where I had gone to catch up on some paperwork. For the five and a half years of Mary Ellen's struggle, whenever Jean Christman, our aide, came to my classroom door with the inevitable white piece of paper indicating a phone call, I'd die a thousand deaths. How I dreaded those phone messages! Now as she approached the door, she again had that dreaded piece of paper. I hastened to the office and called Dr. Gallup, who said, "When you come home, please be aware of the conversation Mary Ellen and I have had. Mary Ellen has spoken freely about her condition and realizes death is imminent. She confided in me that she felt you all had, for these five years, put her on a pedestal, so to speak. She indicated that she was far from pedestal material. I think she wants to talk about this thought."

"I'll be home shortly," I said as I thanked him for coming. He promised to stay in constant contact. He even gave me his mother's phone number, since his own father had just passed away and he often visited with his mother in the evening.

As I reflect upon her words about the pedestal, I don't believe we really and truly put her above all others. What we did do was try, as much as she would permit, to ease her burden by making life a bit easier. We, along with many others, thought she was pretty special, and now that she was sorting out her life, she perhaps felt we had singled her out from all others for a bit of extra-special treatment. We naturally talked about her accomplishments, as did her relatives, friends, and classmates. Perhaps we sometimes embarrased her by "bragging" about her and the efforts she made to be a success in whatever she attempted. Her goals were set and for the most part she achieved them, doing her own thing and being her own person. If that were "putting her on a pedestal," then I guess we were all somewhat guilty.

Mary Ellen also spoke with Dr. Guinan on this day. Being in Boston, three hours from Sheffield, was, I'm certain, a difficult position for Dr. Guinan, who could only communicate with Mary Ellen by phone. I'm also positive, however, that Dr. Guinan, knowing that being at home rather than in the hospital was Mary Ellen's choice, realized the situation now was being handled in the best possible way, with Mary Ellen's wishes uppermost. The conversation between Dr. Guinan and Mary Ellen was brief. "Do you want me to tell you about the final stages of the disease?" Dr. Guinan asked.

Mary Ellen questioned, "Will I feel any pain?"

Dr. Guinan assured her, "No. I promise you'll feel no pain and you will merely go to sleep."

With this, Mary Ellen cried and said, "Goodbye."

When I returned home, Mary Ellen was sleepy and didn't want to talk. She slept a great deal now, and since she wasn't taking in many fluids, Dr. Gallup felt an IV was necessary. That evening, after his hospital rounds at Sharon, he came and spent several hours with us, administering the IV and just talking. He left about midnight, with the promise to stop by the following day. In the meantime, we were to contact Wayne Speyrer so he could monitor the IV and report to Dr. Gallup.

The following day Amy Kissel called from her home on Long Island. She and her mother had just returned from a trip to Chicago and San Francisco. Amy, unaware of the turn of events since she last saw Mary Ellen at the Springfield graduation some two weeks ago, said, "I spoke with her and asked, 'Mary Ellen, how are you? Do you want me to come?' She answered me weakly, 'Yes.'"

Amy, who was going to the campus for a meeting, visited with Mary Ellen that day on her way to Springfield, As Amy left us, she said, "Please call me at the college and let me know how things are."

Family members, too, had been aware of Mary Ellen's condition, so there were many visits and calls. Friends stopped by now frequently just to sit and talk quietly with us and Mary Ellen. Our neighbor, Bertha Newton, Bert to us, stayed during the day, along with Danielle's mom, Priscilla. Both of these nurses took care of Mary Ellen's physical needs. Their dedication these last two or three days, as they bathed her and made her as comfortable as possible, will never be forgotten. I called Wendy and Andy in Bangor, Maine, and Priscilla called Danielle and Mike in Norfolk, Virginia. They all indicated they would leave their homes immediately, arriving in the evening on Thursday. Wendy and Andy came, bringing a little stuffed teddy bear. Mary Ellen perked up when she saw them. Mike and Danielle arrived later in the evening, and again Mary Ellen smiled her happiness. We spoke with Wendy about notifying the Springfield community and Danielle said she would call all the local people who, we felt, would want to say their goodbyes. The advantages of living in a small community now came to the fore as the word spread and our dear friends, who had struggled with us these many years, came to be with us now that the end of the battle was fast approaching.

On Thursday Ken Childs, the minister on the Springfield campus, and his wife, Donna, responded to our phone call. Ken spent about an hour Thursday afternoon talking and praying with Mary Ellen. He assured us he would be able to return any time that we might need him, even though this weekend found the alumni returning to campus. His parting words: "Call me if I can help. Please don't hesitate."

Ken first met Mary Ellen her freshman year as she walked around the campus with Amy. He later said, "My first impression was a young lady full of mischief, kidding around with the people she was with. I had met her, talked with her, and knew her long before I realized she was a cancer patient, or that she had lost her leg for that matter. This was very characteristic, since she never made a big deal about her loss. One of the very remarkable things about Mary Ellen was that she was so matter-of-fact about the loss of her limb. She obviously had her ups and downs but on the whole, she had this philosophy that what was before her had to be dealt with as she went on with her life." Ken continued, "I like to think of Mary Ellen as the athlete playing a sport or a game who, even though she got a few bad calls, wanted to get on with this game of life. She didn't dwell on the bad calls as she and you, her family, tried to normalize life and to go on." Ken concluded as he referred to the last few weeks of her life, "Mary Ellen told me she was getting tired of the treatments and at that point was ready to die. I'm certain Mary Ellen was sustained by the ongoingness of life at this time, since she certainly displayed a spiritual quality now that her life was coming to an end."

216

17

THE FOLLOWING DAY, FRIDAY, JUNE 10, WAS WARM AND SUNNY. Dr. Gallup made his morning visit. My sister and her daughter, Karen, came from New York. During the day there was a steady parade of friends, classmates, and relatives. The outpouring of concern was overwhelming. I don't believe our little community had ever experienced anything like this farewell to Mary Ellen. At Mount Everett, the halls were hushed as the students and teachers went about their routines on a somber note. The committee from the Carnegie Foundation for which Mount Everett was one of the finalists for an exciting three-year grant, voiced its amazement at the concern all had for our family: "Mount Everett is certainly a caring family." The Mount Everett community had indeed exhibited a deep concern these past five years.

I spoke with Dr. Guinan on this morning to keep her informed. She, too, knew it would only be a matter of time, but as she said later, "Perhaps we weren't lucky with this whole situation, but at least no terrible complications surfaced at the end when it really mattered, so Mary Ellen's final hours were peaceful and without pain."

I believe our prayers were answered and Our Lord, in His infinite mercy, took care of Mary Ellen during her final hours on this earth before He and His most Blessed Mother welcomed her into the Kingdom of Heaven for eternity. She had struggled too long and too hard and now deserved to leave this world peacefully.

It would be impossible to mention by name all those who came on Friday, as from mid-morning on there occurred a steady outpouring of love from the community, classmates, and teachers from Mount Everett, Berkshire School, and Springfield College; relatives; friends of Jim Jr.'s and Katherine's. Amy Kissel and Roland Gelinas and many other Springfield friends came. My sister made certain there were plenty of refreshments as she took over the kitchen. Our dear friend Artie Hebert called from

217

California and Mary Ellen smiled at mention of his name. Lisa and Teresa Gulotta called from Arizona. Everyone who had helped to make our struggle easier now came to say their farewells. Katherine, particularly, remained constantly at her sister's bedside, holding her hand and trying to make her as comfortable as possible.

Our sister-in-law, Lorraine, and my brother, Donald, who were Mary Ellen's godparents, spent the day praying with us and for us and for Mary Ellen. In the afternoon, Mary Ellen asked for Aunt Lorraine. When Lorraine came into the room, she asked Mary Ellen, "Do you want me to say the rosary?" Mary Ellen nodded. Lorraine, who is blessed with a beautiful sense of prayer, recited the prayers as we all took part. It was indeed a time filled with awe, as many of the young people gathered around and near the bed listened or prayed with us. We prayed that Our Lady would prepare for Mary Ellen the path to Her Son, Jesus. Twice during the afternoon Lorraine repeated the prayers of the rosary, a very comforting experience.

The youthful congregation in our home, indeed a profound testament to Mary Ellen and to us, filled these last hours with love and caring. These young people, so full of life and so busy with their own lives, came to witness her final hours. They were privileged to observe the dying process in a manner filled with love and prayer, comfort and peace. Death in itself is naturally feared, since we are all so intent on living. Now these young friends, as well as everyone else, prayed with us as we all experienced a peace and a calm, even as we grieved for our loss.

During the day, Mary Ellen gazed at the wall of pictures we referred to as "our rogues' gallery" as she studied all of the family photos from babyhood to teenagers to the present. At one point Katherine cried, "I'm so glad those pictures are there for her."

Occasionally Mary Ellen uttered a few words: "Hurry up, hurry up." And then, as evening came, in a very soft voice, she said a few times, "Okay, okay." Soon after night came almost all of our friends had left but Wendy, Jennifer, Tammy Jervas, Danielle, and Katherine remained with Mary Ellen. Ken Childs and his wife came later in the evening for a last moment. As Ken spoke to Mary

Ellen, she whispered, "Can I stop being brave now?"

Ken, commenting on these words later that evening to Amy, said, "It's as if Mellon is asking permission to give up, to stop the struggle."

A year later Amy, while visiting in Sheffield, remembered these words as she said, "I spent my first semester at graduate school at Columbia reflecting upon this thought as I wrote several papers for my classes. What an incredible thing for Mellon to ask!"

During the night, Priscilla monitored Mary Ellen's vital signs. Dolores, Jim Jr., Jimmy, and I dozed off and on, knowing that before morning Mary Ellen would be welcomed into the Kingdom of Heaven where, as she had said many months before, "At least I'll see my Nanny and Grandpa again." I'm sure they were waiting for her, to welcome her into eternity.

18

❦

SATURDAY, JUNE 11, DAWNED A BEAUTIFUL DAY. AS THE LIGHT of morning brightened, the birds sang and in the field behind our house a doe grazed. An incredibly beautiful dawn! About 5:30, Priscilla indicated that death was fast approaching, and we all gathered to say our final farewell. She perhaps couldn't hear us as we said our goodbyes, but I like to think that as Mary Ellen passed from mortality to immortality, she was aware of her family and close friends. And so we cried our goodbyes, hugging her and leaving her with kisses. Her long struggle had ended and she now began her eternal existence in the "Mansions of the Lord."

Epilogue

Tuesday, June 14, dawned another beautiful day as we prepared to say our last farewell. Our little white church, Our Lady of the Valley, welcomed hundreds of friends and family to take part in the Liturgy of the Word. Never had it seen such a crowd! The Mount Everett High School was closed for the day in Mary Ellen's honor. Chairs had been placed outside, and our dear friend, Joe Seward, had wired speakers so everyone on the lawn could share in the service. A good friend, Sally Cook, remembered this day as she wrote:

> *So much you have been in my thoughts—as you well know, the whole town's. We will forever remember that service at Our Lady of the Valley— the caring and love of the whole town was right there.... We have all tried to put ourselves in your place. And I am certain that none of us feel we could have managed these last years as you have—with such dignity, reality, and generosity. You and Mary Ellen have touched all our lives deeply for a long time now—whether we have verbalized it or not. Sometimes we have asked; sometimes we were hesitant. But always our hearts went out to each of you. Mary Ellen and you have given us so very much. Our lives will all be lived a little differently; a little more carefully and with more appreciation for life itself and with a little more love. In all that has been taken away, so much has been given, that energy and purpose never dies.*

Channing Murdock, owner of the ski area, Butternut Basin, also recalled this day:

> *Dear Folks:*
> *I'm terribly sorry I didn't get to catch up with any of you at the church service for Mary Ellen. The overwhelming support of your friends only highlights the very special feelings which Mary Ellen and her family have generated over the years. If only more families were able to love and relate to themselves and their friends as you have, the world would be a much healthier and happier place.*
> *My relatively brief acquaintance with Mary Ellen has certainly enriched my life. I am glad to have had the opportunity to know her and to feel that I could be part of the large group of her friends who gathered*

in her honor in Sheffield.

My thoughts are with each of you, with the hope that you can maintain the strength that you have shown over the past difficult years.

As she was loved in life, so, too, was she loved in death. The beauty of the service and those who came to join us eased our sorrow. Finally we bid our farewell as the choir, filled with many nonmembers of our church who wanted to play a part in the service, sang the final hymn, so appropriate, "On Eagles' Wings."

And He will raise you up on eagles' wings
Bear you on the breath of dawn,
Make you shine like the sun,
And hold you in the palm of His hand.

Later in the day, students from Springfield College, Mount Everett, and Berkshire School, as well as friends from Boston, joined family, friends, and neighbors at our home to again reminisce and to remember Mary Ellen in a lighter atmosphere. She would have approved of the gathering as her many friends mingled with family. And now, the tapestry threads, woven together, complete the imagery begun in November 1982. All who gathered at our home on this June afternoon, as well as all who came to say goodbye at our church that morning, will forever be a part of Mary Ellen's struggle, since they are etched into this weave and texture of threads—her tapestry of courage.

During that afternoon, the Mount Everett softball team, coached by Kelly Milan was to play a crucial game to determine whether or not the team would go to the Western Massachusetts Division III finals.

A news article written by Howard Herman and appearing in the *Berkshire Eagle* on Wednesday, June 15, 1988, told the story.

Chicopee—. . . The Eagles rode the strong right arm of Sue Carpenter to an emotional 3-2 eight-inning upset of two-time defending state champ Smith Academy at Szot Park. The come-from-behind win physically and emotionally drained coach Kelly Milan and her Eagles, who had attended the funeral of former Eagle player Mary Ellen Welch before boarding the bus to Chicopee. Welch, a close friend of Milan's and the team's, died Saturday of bone cancer.

It was not a down Mount Everett team that played yesterday, despite the overriding emotions.

'Anyone who knew Mary Ellen would know she wouldn't want us to be down, she wouldn't want us to be depressed,' said Milan, full of mixed emotions after the game. 'If we came here hanging our heads, she would be upset with us. So we didn't, we came with them up.'

. . . The Eagles wore black armbands in memory of Welch, who was not only a former Mount Everett player, but also godmother to Milan's two-year-old son, Corey. Going right from the funeral to the game made for a potentially difficult situation. It was a situation that the Eagles handled with dignity.

'So many of us were there [at the funeral] today, that we knew what we had to do,' said Carpenter. 'We all waited on the bus and put our armbands on together. We just knew that inside we had to be awesome today.'

As the game ended, the coach of Smith Academy, Sherry Webb, a Springfield College graduate who had also been at the funeral, summed up the outcome of the game when she said to Kelly, "You had an extra player on the field today."

Mary Ellen's memory will forever be perpetuated by awards and scholarships:

The Mary Ellen Welch Memorial Scholarship, awarded each year to a graduate of Mount Everett Regional School, Sheffield, Massachusetts.

The Sheffield Kiwanis Club has named one of its scholarships the Mary Ellen Welch Scholarship. It will be awarded to a graduate of Mount Everett Regional School or Monument Mountain Regional School, Great Barrington, Massachusetts.

The Mary Ellen Welch Softball Award, given to a member of the Mount Everett team each year who displays that certain quality of spunk which Mary Ellen possessed.

The Mary Ellen Welch Softball Award, given to a member of the Berkshire School team who best exemplifies the dedication, sportsmanship, and courage displayed by Mary Ellen.

A Memorial Garden prominently displaying a teddy bear marker on the campus of Springfield College, given in her memory by her classmates, the Class of 1989.

The proceeds from this book will be used to inaugurate a scholarship or some other award at Springfield College, Springfield, Massachusetts, in Mary Ellen's memory.

About Osteogenic Sarcoma

A discussion of the disease follows, with excerpts from a term paper Mary Ellen wrote for her Pediatric Rehabilitation course at Springfield College in April 1987. I believe the paper will prove interesting and informative and may clarify many medical terms discussed in this book.

Osteogenic sarcoma, also known as osteosarcoma, is the most common form of bone cancer in children (*Young People with Cancer*, p. 12). The tumors most commonly appear on the ends of bones. Such bones that are usually affected are the upper arm [humerus] and the leg [tibia and femur]. Osteogenic sarcoma usually occurs between the ages of ten and twenty-five, and is also more common in males than females (*Young People with Cancer*, p. 12).

As with most cancers, the cause of osteosarcoma is unknown. However, the connection between the age of the young person and the location of the primary tumor can give some information as to the relation of increased cell division and function (Dahlin, p. 191).

223

Young people with this type of cancer usually complain of constant pain and at times swelling, which usually the child may blame on an injury. Another common symptom of osteosarcoma is a sudden growth spurt (*Young People with Cancer*, p. 12). If I may bring some personal insight into this paper, I never had a sudden growth spurt and I am not a male. However, I did have a pain in my knee; therefore, the symptoms may not always relate to every case. Diagnosing the disease can be difficult, as osteosarcoma may be easily confused (when looking at an X-ray) with a number of different things, such as infections, previous effects of an injury, or benign tumors. The only way to confirm the disease is to perform a biopsy. Because the disease is known to spread [metastasize] to other parts of the body, most commonly the lungs, chest X-rays, CAT scans of the chest, and bone scans may also be done before any treatment begins (*Young People with Cancer*).

Treatment should be started immediately after the diagnosis has been made. It is important that treatment be given at a center that has an experienced staff and the equipment to supply the most effective forms of treatment. Such a center is the Dana-Farber Cancer Institute/Children's Hospital in Boston, Massachusetts (*Young People with Cancer*, p. 13). The first phase is the surgical treatment of the primary tumor, which entails the amputation or "wide surgical excision [limb salvage] of the affected limb." Limb salvage is done only at the discretion of the surgeon (Goorin, p. 16). As soon as the surgery is done and the patient has made sufficient recovery [usually two weeks from surgery], the next phase of treatment, either chemotherapy [treatment of cancer with special drugs that destroy cancer cells, most often taken through a needle inserted into a vein, called an intravenous or IV for short] or radiation [treatment of cancer with X-rays or rays from other radioactive sources] is begun.

Some types of cancer treatment programs have been established, but research for more effective treatment is constantly underway. With osteosarcoma, the patient may be treated under the direction of a protocol, a general treatment plan used by a group of hospitals for this specific type of cancer. The protocol is designed to set up the ideal type, frequency, and duration of treatment (*Young People with Cancer*, p. 14). The protocol for osteosarcoma, as set up by the Dana-Farber in Boston and other collaborating hospitals, involves six different drugs: Methotrexate, Adriamycin, Bleomycin, Cytoxan, Actinomycin D, and Cisplatin (Goorin, p. 4).

As with any new experience, there are always many questions that may arise. One major question frequently asked is, "What are the risks and what are the benefits of such a study protocol?" The major risks to the chemotherapy patient is the concern of toxicities of the drugs used. For example, the drug Methotrexate may cause nausea, depression in blood count, kidney damage, and mouth sores (Goorin, p. 4). Each of the other drugs mentioned has its own list of toxicities or side effects that must be spelled out to the patient and family. The side effects may not all happen since each patient is different. Most side effects are not permanent and will improve once the drugs are stopped (*Young People with Cancer*, p. 21).

Another form of treatment used in the battle against cancer is radiation. However, radiation is not used very often with osteosarcoma patients due to its poor success record. The basic ideas of radiation [treatment by high energy X-ray] are simple: X-rays, radium, and other sources of ionizing radiation are used to destroy cancer cells before they divide. Radiation may be used alone or in conjunction with surgery or chemo or both.

Living with cancer is very difficult, not knowing what each trip to the doctor will bring. Perhaps the best treatment for anyone with osteosarcoma would be to make his or her life as "normal" as possible and to take one day at a time.

The chart that follows illustrates the thirteen month protocol followed by patients with osteosarcoma (Goorin, p. 39).

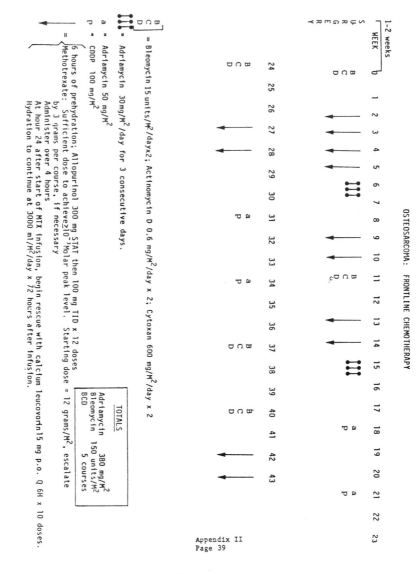

B
C = Bleomycin 15 units/M²/dayx2; Actinomycin D 0.6 mg/M²/day x 2; Cytoxan 600 mg/M²/day x 2
D

a = Adriamycin 30mg/M²/day for 3 consecutive days.

a = Adriamycin 50 mg/M²
p = CDDP 100 mg/M²

= 6 hours of prehydration: Allopurinol 300 mg STAT then 100 mg TID x 12 doses

= Methotrexate: Sufficient dose to achieve ≥10⁻³ Molar peak level. Starting dose = 12 grams/M², escalate by 3 grams per course, if necessary. Administer over 4 hours. At hour 24 after start of MTX infusion, begin rescue with calcium leucovorin 15 mg p.o. Q 6H x 10 doses. Hydration to continue at 3000 ml/M²/day x 72 hours after infusion.

TOTALS	
Adriamycin	380 mg/M²
Bleomycin	150 units/M²
BCD	5 courses

Appendix II
Page 39

Protocol for Osteogenic Sarcoma Patients

Bibliography

Dahlin, D.C. *Osteosarcoma of Bone and a Consideration of Prognostic Variables*, Cancer Treatment Rep. (1978), Vol 62, pp. 189-92.

Goorin, Allen M., M.D. "Multi-Institutional Controlled Trial of Adjuvant Chemotherapy in the Treatment of Osteosarcoma" Sidney Farber Cancer Institute, Boston, MA, 1981, pp. 4-16, 39.

Stolov, Walter C. *Handbook of Severe Disability: A Text for Rehabilitation Counselors, Other Vocational Practitioners, and Allied Health Professionals* (Library of Congress), pp. 17; 1, 172, 180-9.

Eating Hints: Recipes and Tips for Better Nutrition During Cancer Treatment, U.S. Department of Human Services, National Cancer Institute, Maryland, 1982, pp. 1-2.

Young People with Cancer: A Handbook for Parents, U.S. Department of Human Services, National Cancer Institute, Maryland, 1983, pp. 10-25.